Printed by CreateSpace, an Amazon Company

ISBN-13: 978-1540666185
(CreateSpace-Assigned)
ISBN-10: 1540666182

A Rough Season

A Memoir

Martha Warriner Jarrett

This memoir is dedicated to my doctor, Sam Raman, for saving my life; to Magic Johnson, for showing everyone that a man with HIV can still play basketball—and so much more; to my wonderful husband, Ronald, for saving my life, and for helping me to start living again; and to the roughly 156,000 Americans who are living with HIV but don't know it.

Chapter 1

In this country today, there are around 1.2 million people living with HIV. Roughly 156,000 of them don't know they are infected. Until two years ago, when I tested positive for HIV at age seventy, I was one of those people. This is my story.

About two years ago, my husband Ronald became concerned about the really bad headaches I'd been having for several days, so he took me to a Kaiser urgent-care facility three different times over the course of a couple of days. The third time they said my blood pressure was 200/130 (extremely high), which meant that I was in Stage 3 hypertensive crisis and required emergency care. Because of the state I was in, they told Ronald I'd have to go to the emergency room. But I fought him when he tried to get me out of the car. Then they stuck me in an ambulance and took me off to the emergency room. I threw up all over the EMTs, then I fought with them. Not normal behavior for me by any stretch of the imagination. And, of course, I remember none of this.

By the time Ronald followed the ambulance, parked the car, and got in to the emergency room, they already had me on a breathing tube. I was in acute respiratory distress. That scared him to death. But that's how I stayed for the next four days.

Ronald was afraid I was going to die. I guess I almost did. He visited me every day, although I wasn't aware he was there. He even brought some of my favorite Dave Koz smooth jazz CDs and played them for me while I was unconscious. It must have worked. After four days, I woke up (although it took a few more days before I became aware of my surroundings).

In the hospital, the doctor told Ronald that I'd tested HIV positive, but not much more. They tested him and he was negative. When he told me I'd tested HIV positive, shortly after I regained consciousness, I couldn't have been more shocked. I simply couldn't believe it. After all, I'd never done anything to get HIV or AIDS. I've since read my hospital records, and they indicate that the doctor spent a lot of time talking to Ronald and me about HIV, but neither of us remembers any such conversation. That would be par for the course for me—I was pretty much out of it at the time—but there's no reason why Ronald wouldn't have remembered. So I think we can safely assume the conversations never took place.

At the time, I was a seventy-year-old white heterosexual woman, which means I was one of the least likely people on the planet to be infected. I had a successful legal career. I was happily married to my second husband, Alan, for nearly twenty-five years, and I was never unfaithful. But there it was. I was HIV positive. Or so the doctors said. I was in denial. I didn't want to believe it. What was happening to me? It wasn't real.

While I was in the medically induced coma, the nurses were crying on Ronald's shoulder because they didn't think my doctor knew what she was doing. Apparently, the hospital agreed, because they brought in a specialist to consult, but Kaiser wouldn't pay him to take over my case. In the meantime, the nurse who'd been the most upset about my case had been assigned to a different patient, and my husband couldn't even talk to her anymore.

After four days, they unhooked me from the ventilator and I woke up, although I still don't remember any of this. I was able to get out of bed—with help—and go to the bathroom. After they moved me from intensive care into a regular room, my husband slept the last two nights in the room with me.

When I was ready to leave the hospital, they sent me to a rehab facility. Because the hospital didn't have an ambulance available, they asked Ronald to drive me. They gave him directions, and he tried to find the place. The first thing I remember after I woke up was Ronald trying to find it on a dark, rainy night. We were new to Bakersfield, California, where we'd just moved, and he got hopelessly lost, so he did the only thing he knew to do: he took me home and put me to bed. When he went out to the car to get something, he made me promise not to get up. But, obstinate to the core (I'm a Capricorn), when I needed to go to the bathroom, I got up. Of course, I fell and hit my head on something. When Ronald came back in, there was blood everywhere. He didn't leave my side until the next morning. I vaguely remember this, but my memory of it is out of place and context. What I remember is falling when I was coming up the stairs, but we lived in a one-floor apartment.

The next morning, he took me back to the hospital. They finally had an ambulance available, so they took me to the rehab facility, with Ronald following. The place where they took me was old—linoleum floors, old plumbing, and so on—but it was clean, the staff was very nice, and the food was certainly edible. When I got there, they put me in a room with one other woman. She spent the day yelling at nothing in particular. The staff apologized and told me they were looking for another room for me. Thankfully, they found one before dinnertime, because the yelling had gotten really annoying. Sleeping, which was all I wanted to do, was difficult. I still didn't understand why I was there.

There were four beds in my new room. And although the women were friendly, there didn't seem to be a reason for any of them to be there other than old age and an inability to care for themselves. I was afraid that might be where I was heading. Of course, the nurses told me not to get out of bed and to ring if I needed to go to the bathroom. True to form, however, I went by myself. Fortunately, there were plenty of things I could hold on to all the way, so I didn't fall again. A few days later, in the middle of the night when I couldn't sleep, I got up and wandered the halls, talking to any of the other patients who were awake. Again, I made it back to bed safely.

I spent four or five days doing little more than sleeping and eating. I didn't even want to read a book, which was highly unusual for the voracious reader in me. Ronald visited me every day, and I'd wait impatiently for him to arrive. Apparently, I didn't have my phone with me because I didn't have any way to contact him to find out when he'd get there. He brought me clothes from Walmart so I could wear something other than a hospital gown. The first batch was stolen before I'd even had a chance to wear any of them. So he brought me some more.

While I was in rehab, I had a visit from Alan's daughter, Maddy, along with a couple of my friends, Dick and Monica. One afternoon there was a soft knock on the door. I looked up and there were the three of them. We chatted for a few minutes, and Maddy told me she'd been researching nursing homes and had found one in LA that was really nice. It even had a chef. Wouldn't I like to move there? Without thinking, I said, "Sure," not realizing she hadn't run her plan by Ronald first. And it didn't occur to me to tell her that I was supposed to go home in a few days. I'd also forgotten that she has a way of thinking she runs the world. She's like a tenacious mother who thinks she can decide what's best for everyone, even those who aren't her children. She'd even cleared the move with the facility—they said I could leave whenever I wanted to. But, of course, she didn't realize I hadn't really meant that I wanted to be moved.

Then we started talking about my HIV diagnosis, which was still pretty new to me. Maddy stated unequivocally that I must have gotten it from her father, my late husband, Alan. I wanted to slap her for being so disrespectful of him. I now know that the suggestion actually came from Monica (which, unfortunately, also sounds like something she would say). I've only spoken to her once since then.

When the visit was over, and I was so tired I could hardly keep my eyes open, Ronald followed Maddy into the hall. I guess that was when the shit really hit the fan. He accused her of trying to kidnap me. After arguing for several minutes, he apparently threatened to kill her. I laughed when I heard about it, but the facility called the police. When they showed up, they listened to both sides of the story, then took Ronald outside and told him they'd checked and knew he didn't own a gun, and to call them if he needed any help and they'd "take care of her" for trying to kidnap his wife. Fortunately, he's never needed their help.

That little episode cooled my relationship with Maddy for quite a while. When Ronald finally calmed down, I assured him it was just Maddy being Maddy. It was only recently that I found out how she'd found me. Ronald had been so wound up worrying about me that he hadn't called anybody to tell them I was in the hospital. At least that's what I thought until I started writing this book and asking questions. It turns out he'd called Dick and a few other close friends and told them what was going on. But even then, Ronald had no idea that Dick and Maddy knew each other. I'd asked Dick to help her out some years before with a real estate problem. So, obviously, Dick had called Maddy after he'd gotten the call from Ronald.

I couldn't just ignore Maddy. After all, she was the mother of three of my grandchildren. And while I never really thought of her as my real daughter, I certainly thought of her children as my grandchildren.

I went home from the rehab facility a few days after Maddy's visit. Of course, that derailed her plan to move me to a nicer facility. As I realized later, after I was back on my feet, she apparently thought I'd be in some kind of a facility for the rest of my life. The first time I saw her, a few weeks later, her mouth dropped open in surprise as I walked out to greet her.

Once I was home, it took two or three weeks for me to pretty much get back on my feet, although I still needed Ronald's help for another month or so. I couldn't even get in and out of the bathtub without his help, and I certainly didn't feel strong enough to stand up and take a shower. We had the apartment maintenance people remove the sliding doors around the tub and store them someplace. I felt like some kind of an invalid, being pushed around in a wheelchair. Even worse was using the walker. I mostly stayed in bed sleeping for the first couple of weeks. I had plenty of time to wonder how this awful thing had happened.

Slowly, it began to dawn on me that Maddy had to be right: I must have gotten HIV from Alan. There just wasn't any other plausible explanation. But while my mind acknowledged it, I guess my heart didn't, so I rarely thought about it, much less talked about it. Nor could I think about where Alan had gotten it. In the back of my mind, I knew it meant he must have been unfaithful, but I wasn't ready to face that possibility yet. It was too bitter a pill to swallow; it took months before I could confront it. I'd certainly never suspected there was anyone else. I still think it must have been nothing more than a onetime fling, but I could be wrong. And as I delved deeper into the whole HIV thing, I came to realize that Alan might well have gotten it from another man. It's fairly rare for a woman to give it to a man. It took me more than a year to really acknowledge that he'd not only given it to me, but that he'd been unfaithful—and to be able to talk about any of it.

I've forgiven Alan for giving me HIV because I'm sure he didn't know he had it. But I haven't been able to forgive him for being unfaithful. If I'd known about it before he died, it would have ended our marriage. It seems to me that the women who stay in a marriage once they find out their husbands have been unfaithful are the ones who suspected all along that it was happening. It's the women like me, who never suspected anything, who leave.

Knowing now that he gave me HIV has changed everything. It's pretty much trashed over twenty-five years of otherwise wonderful memories. I still have the memories, but when I think about them, there's a tinge of anger and bitterness. I can't believe he was so stupid as to have had unprotected sex.

When I finally came home, my routine didn't really change. After a few days, a physical therapist showed up at home and gave me some exercises to get me back on my feet and to build my stamina and coordination. Ronald got some protein powder at the health food store and started making milkshakes for me to help me put the weight I'd lost back on.

It was a strange experience not to be able to walk without help, but I guess the therapy worked. Although I progressed slowly—at least that's how it felt to me—after a few weeks, I was pretty much back on my feet.

About two weeks after I got home, we went out for Christmas dinner with the kids, and with our son-in-law's parents. I think we went to Coco's—about the only thing open on Christmas Day. Ronald pushed me in the wheel chair. I had to use the handicap ramp to get inside.

After I'd been home for several weeks, and after the latest in a series of crying jags, Ronald asked me if I was going to just lie around crying and feeling sorry for myself. But I didn't know what else to do. I was in a fog. It felt like I was drowning in a deep mysterious pool. There was no place for me to go in Bakersfield to deal with my grief. I've always liked long walks on the beach—it's what I used to do to regain my equilibrium whenever I was upset or in pain. But there's no beach in Bakersfield, or even much of a lake. And the Kern River is either dry, or underground. So I had no place to turn but inward—not the best place to go when you're in pain. And I was still in denial about the HIV diagnosis. To say I was scared would be an understatement. I was terrified. My life was shattered. I was afraid I might never recover.

But Ronald and his daughter had done some research, and they told me that there were two more tests I would need to take to confirm that I didn't have HIV.

They'd checked around and determined that Planned Parenthood was probably the best place to get the other two tests. Who knew? I'm not one of those people who thinks Planned Parenthood is just about abortions. But HIV and AIDS? So, I made an appointment and had the second test done. Much to my dismay, it also came back positive. This was beginning to look really bad. When the third test also came back positive, I couldn't believe it. I started to cry again. How had this happened? I still had no idea.

The counselor at Planned Parenthood spent a long time with Ronald and me, talking about what my diagnosis meant and how I might have acquired HIV. I told her I didn't know. They tested Ronald and, again, the results were negative. I obviously hadn't gotten it from him.

I'm a lawyer so I'm used to dealing with tough issues, but when it's about yourself, it's a whole different ball game. All this time, I was still feeling sorry for myself, and I was still scared. What was going on? How would I cope with all this bad news? How could I handle all these medical problems? What was next? Ronald tried to cheer me up, but didn't help.

On the other hand, maybe it really did help. If he hadn't been there, spotting problems when they came up, I'm quite sure I wouldn't have survived. I was that sick. But I couldn't see it myself. I had no idea anything was wrong.

I still can't remember much of anything that happened during the two months before I ended up in the emergency room. I remember Thanksgiving dinner. Ronald and I went to a wonderful buffet at the Padre Hotel, an old establishment in downtown Bakersfield that had been recently renovated. The meal was perfect—all the traditional Thanksgiving goodies, plus a few more exotic ones, like crab legs and raw oysters—and very romantic.

And I remember going somewhere by myself late one afternoon. I realized that I had turned in the wrong direction, so I made a U-turn. The sun was in my eyes, and when I turned, I ran over the median and damaged the undercarriage of the car. I stopped at the nearest service station and called the Auto Club. The guy came, straightened out some stuff under the car, and told me it was fine. But by then, I had no idea where I was or how to get home (we'd only been in Bakersfield for a couple of weeks). So, I called Ronald's daughter, and she guided me home. A couple of days later, the car started making funny noises again, so we took it to the dealer. The damage was much more severe than we'd originally thought (about $1,500 worth). Things were starting to go wrong, but I couldn't see it yet.

The other thing I remember was crashing into the bedroom door in the middle of the night when I got up to go to the bathroom. It didn't feel like I'd done any damage, other than a small cut above my left eye, but Ronald insisted on taking me to the emergency room, just in case. They did all kinds of tests. I didn't have a concussion, but before they sent me home, they started questioning Ronald to determine whether he'd hit me. Fortunately, Ronald's ex-wife is an expert in domestic violence, so he knew immediately where the questions were leading, and he also knew how to answer them so that it quickly became obvious that he wasn't the culprit. And he also told them about other things that had been happening to me that made him think I was rapidly descending into dementia.

After that scare, life went back to normal—or so I thought. A month later, I woke up in the hospital from a medically induced coma.

I'd like my story to serve as a wake-up call to everyone. The test for HIV is simple and it isn't expensive. There's even a home test now available called OraQuick, and it costs about forty dollars. So please get tested. Even if you don't think you could have been exposed—without getting tested, you don't know for sure. And since HIV/AIDS has become a manageable disease—kind of like diabetes—people seem to have become complacent. Please don't be. It's still a nasty and sometimes fatal disease. The epidemic is definitely NOT over.

But, more important, I hope my story also serves as a wake-up call for doctors. If you have a patient who is sick, no matter what age, and you can't figure out what's wrong no matter how hard you've tried, test them for HIV. My late husband died because no one thought to test him, probably because he was in his late seventies at the time. I nearly died because the same thing happened to me. Don't let this happen to you or anyone else. There are so many indicators for HIV, it simply doesn't make sense for doctors not to test for it.

Chapter 2

My husband Ronald and I met more than thirty years ago, when I was a young attorney, and he was a lawyer in the legal department of Getty Oil Company, where we both worked. He was in the Tulsa office; I was in the Los Angeles one. I'd gone to Houston for a seminar on the regulations that governed oil and gasoline supplies and prices at the time, so that's how I ended up in Houston a couple of weeks before Christmas in 1978.

At the end of the first day of the seminar, I went to dinner with Ronald and a group of other attorneys and accountants from the Tulsa office of Getty. At the end of dinner, as everyone started to go their separate ways, Ronald asked me if I'd like to join him for a drink. He was an attractive, light-skinned African American who in those days looked a lot like the baseball legend, Reggie Jackson. Plus, he had a wonderful smile. He seemed nice, and he worked for the same company I did, so I said yes.

We went to the revolving bar at the top of the Hyatt Regency and took a seat where we could see the lights of Houston. We talked for a couple of hours about ourselves and our families—he was married with a young daughter; I was married but had no children—and our respective marital problems. Neither of us was in the kind of marriage that was easy to leave. There was no infidelity or abuse or anything like that. Mine just wasn't living up to my expectations of marriage. Finally, he walked me back to my room, he kissed me on the cheek, and we said good night. The next day, when I got on the plane back to LA, I could already tell my marriage was in even more trouble than I'd thought.

It didn't take long for me to figure out that the attraction was mutual. I visited the Tulsa office a couple of times a month during that period, and Ronald and I generally had lunch or dinner on the two or three days I was in town. He was supposed to pick me up at the Tulsa airport late one Sunday night, but my plane was delayed by fog in LA for several hours. When we were finally cleared for takeoff, we could hear the plane ahead of us gun its engines. Our pilot never even slowed down. He just followed the first plane and off we went.

When I got to Tulsa, Ronald wasn't waiting at the airport. Because it was late Sunday night, and he had a family, that didn't surprise me. I just took a cab to the hotel. When I got to the office the next morning, I called him from an office in another department. He was surprised I was even in Tulsa. The airline had told him my plane had never left LA.

We went to lunch that day and probably to dinner the next night. After several evenings of such dinners, over the course of a few weeks, we were dancing one night in the hotel bar. We looked at each other. He took my hand and led me out the door and up to my room. We undressed each other and fell onto the bed. The sex was spectacular, but he had a wife waiting at home, so he left in the wee small hours.

When I was back in LA, we spent hours on the phone every day. After a month or so, I decided it was finally time to leave my husband, Paul. I felt really bad about it because I couldn't really say what was wrong with the marriage. Years later, I finally figured out that—like my father—he was just *too* nice. Like a lot of women, there was a part of me that liked "bad boys." But when I tried dating a few of them, I found that the bad boy part wore thin pretty fast.

I told Paul that I was leaving one Friday evening. By Saturday afternoon, I'd packed and left. A friend from law school offered me a place to stay and that's where I went.

After I got settled, I started looking for an apartment. I found one in the Brentwood area of Los Angeles, but it wouldn't be available for almost a month. I didn't think I could stay with my girlfriend for that long, so I found a long-term motel close to the beach in Santa Monica and moved in the following weekend. It was pretty much a run-down dump, but I stayed there for the next two weeks. The final straw was when the lettuce I'd bought to make salads froze in the refrigerator. The cockroaches weren't too appealing either.

A friend of mine at work said he was moving out of his apartment and I could use his old place until the end of that month. I jumped at it. What an improvement!

During this period, I rendezvoused with Ronald one weekend in Houston. Once the conference we were attending was over, we moved to a nice motel. We spent a lot of the weekend in bed. But we also drove to Galveston one afternoon and walked on the beach, which has always been one of my favorite things to do (in good or bad times). And we explored the restaurant scene. We took the same flight back to Tulsa, where I was expected on Monday morning. Although we tried to be careful, we ran into my boss from LA in the Tulsa airport. I had no idea he'd be in town. We told him we'd run into each other on the plane—not a very plausible story, but the best we could come up with on the spur of the moment. He never said anything to either of us. Neither did anyone else, but I guess our relationship had become an open secret.

Around this time, Ronald asked me to marry him. Although I was madly in love with him, I told him it was too soon and asked him to slow down a bit. The next time the subject came up was probably a month or so later. Still not very long. Although I knew I wanted to marry him more than anything, I still hesitated. I guess I was worried that I didn't know him well enough; that I might regret a hasty decision. But I didn't do a very good job of explaining myself to him. He thought I just wanted to play around before I settled down after my divorce. We continued seeing each other, and the sex continued to be off the charts, but something just didn't feel right. Rather than confronting the issue and talking about it, however, I think I was trying too hard to hold on.

By this time, Ronald had started looking for a job in California. When he got one, it was at Occidental

Petroleum in Bakersfield—not my idea of someplace I wanted to live. But he hadn't talked to me about it before he accepted it, which I thought was a little strange. When it was time for him to drive to California, I met him in Albuquerque to help him with the driving—although he never let me drive. When he met me at the Albuquerque Airport, I arrived at the gate next to the one where Ted Kennedy and his entourage had arrived at about the same time. Ronald was upset at the way Kennedy's security people were shoving people around, including me.

Ronald had a funny little red Dodge Colt that didn't have much power. We started driving right after the Fourth of July, so it was really hot coming across the desert. But whenever we turned the air-conditioning on, the car overheated. We spent most of the trip with it turned off and all the windows open.

The first night on the road, we stopped in Kingman, Arizona. I don't remember which motel we stayed in, but I do remember eating an outstanding steak. The second night, I think we stayed in Barstow. All this time, things were feeling really weird. Again, I think I was trying too hard to hold on. And, again, we didn't talk about it. We got to my apartment the following afternoon.

He spent the night with me, then drove on to Bakersfield the next morning.

One day a month or so later, I was in the Tulsa office talking to Ronald's former secretary. She told me Ronald and his wife had sold their house in Tulsa, and his wife was packing to move out to Bakersfield, and wasn't that wonderful? Not exactly. I know the horror I was feeling must have shown on my face. I went into an empty office, closed the door, and called him. I was livid. I read him the riot act in as quiet a voice as I could manage, but I'm sure his secretary still got an earful.

This courtship had been the most romantic thing I'd ever experienced. Then, one day a few months later, it ended as quickly as it had begun. It wasn't long after he moved to Bakersfield when Ronald showed up at my apartment one Saturday afternoon for a scheduled date. We had tickets that night for a Bette Midler concert at the Greek Theatre. He knew I was really looking forward to it. But he picked that day to tell me he'd decided to stay with his wife. There was no conversation about our relationship or why he'd changed his mind about marrying me. Just good-bye. I felt like the bottom had dropped out of my world. I couldn't even speak. I just let him leave. I called a friend and gave her the tickets. Then I spent the afternoon sitting on the floor, in tears.

It was months before I recovered enough to even talk to Ronald again. He started calling me once in a while when he was in LA, and I would visit him in his hotel room. The sex was the same as always, but nothing else was left, or so it seemed. One night he came to my place. When he started to lead me into the bedroom, I stopped him. I told him that if he wanted to resume our relationship, that would be great. But if not, he should leave. He left.

It took several months for me to recover enough to even go out with another man. Although I eventually started dating again, and even had a few long-term relationships, I'd about given up when I meet Alan.

Chapter 3

I met Alan a couple of years after Ronald walked out. I thought he was the man of my dreams. I guess he was for a time. He was tall and handsome, with big brown eyes and a full head of gray hair, although he was only in his late forties. We met at a relationship workshop, an offshoot of est Training, one of the self-help programs popular in the eighties. One of the first exercises involved staring into another person's eyes and saying whether you did or didn't trust him or her, or weren't sure. Alan was the only person in the room I said I *didn't* trust. I found out later he thought he'd had a neutral expression on his face that night, but that wasn't the way I saw it. I came to call it his storm-cloud face. It would show up periodically when he was upset or angry about something.

Fortunately, he pursued me for the rest of the workshop and got me to change my mind. We exchanged phone numbers, and he said he would call me. Several days after the workshop ended, when I hadn't heard from him, I called him and invited him to go with me to a guest seminar for the est Training. It had done a lot for me, and

I wanted him to have the same positive experience. He confessed that he'd lost my phone number and probably wouldn't have tried to find it, but he was happy I'd called. We met before the seminar began. I was waiting outside where people drove in. I spotted him immediately in his tiny yellow Honda Civic.

He didn't enroll in the Training that evening at the guest seminar, but he did follow me home afterward. We enjoyed a glass of wine and eventually ended up in bed. He moved in with me a month or two later. We lived together for about four years before we got married.

He clearly had issues with marriage. He was thirteen years older than me and had the typical concern that he would die and leave me alone when I was still a young woman. I responded in the usual way—it's better to have ten good years than no years at all. Also, he'd just come out of a very bitter divorce, felt his ex-wife had taken him to the cleaners and that I, as a family law attorney, might do the same thing. I assured him that, as someone with my own business, I wasn't about to marry him without a pre-nuptial agreement that would protect *my* assets if we ever got a divorce. But he always resented the money he had to pay his ex-wife for spousal support.

Knowing from my family law experience that the amount he was ordered to pay was relatively small, but being unable to change his mind, I finally sent him to a friend who practiced family law and she finally convinced him that he shouldn't try to modify the amount because that would just put him in danger of having his ex ask that her support be *increased*. But that didn't keep him from resenting it. He finally started paying her twice a year. At least then he didn't have to get upset every month when he wrote the check.

Just when I'd given up on his ever asking me to marry him, he proposed one evening while we were having dinner at the Rose Café in Venice. We were due to leave in a few days on a trip to Albuquerque for the Hot Air Balloon Festival, and planned a side trip to Santa Fe. When we'd been in Santa Fe together a couple of years earlier, he'd spotted a ring and had me try it on. At the time, it had freaked me out. Was he proposing? No. He just liked the ring. I sometimes teased him that he only married me so he could buy me that ring. When he finally proposed, he wanted to go back to Santa Fe and get the ring, and he wanted to buy the diamond before we left.

But first he wanted to make sure I'd say yes. As if there was ever any doubt.

He bought the diamond the next day at the Jewelry Mart in downtown LA and brought it home in one of those little manila jeweler's envelopes. When he opened it, he carefully unfolded the tissue paper. No diamond. We both just about had heart failure. Then he turned the envelope upside down, and out it fell. Talk about a big sigh of relief!

We had a wonderful trip. One of the subcontractors Alan managed in Albuquerque had a hot-air balloon, so we were able to go up for a ride. What a thrill. When the propane burner was turned on, all the dogs on the ground started barking at us as we passed by overhead. Other than that, it was completely silent as we floated along.

But it was the Balloon Festival itself that was the best part. The color of all those balloons rising into the air at the same time during the mass ascension each morning was just amazing. As far as I was concerned, it beat the Rose Parade by a mile. Of course, I somehow lost the full roll of pictures I'd taken of the colorful scene.

The next day we drove to Santa Fe and bought the ring. It was a wide gold band inlaid with lapis lazuli, with the diamond mounted in the middle, and a narrow gold band on one edge, like an engagement ring and wedding ring together. We left the diamond with the jeweler so he could make up the ring. A couple of weeks later, it arrived at my office in the mail, and we were officially engaged.

We got married about a year later. It was a small do-it-yourself wedding in the recreation room of the condo where we were living. Neither of us had much money back then, so Alan barbecued chicken wings, and a friend brought a fruit platter for the reception. At that time, I was in practice for myself and belonged to a barter service, so I was able to trade my legal services for lots of other things. I used my credits for a DJ and a beautiful wedding cake with fresh flowers all over it. It was a special day.

Alan's Aunt Jean from Las Vegas came for the wedding. She'd been like a second mother to him after his mom died when he was in high school. His son David was his best man; and his daughter, Maddy, and her boyfriend came. My best friend from law school, Mary Jo, was my matron of honor. My brother Dick and his wife, Wanda, were there, too.

We were flying to Hawaii the next day, so we spent our wedding night in a hotel near the LA airport. We'd rented a condo in Poipu Beach on Kauai for a week, and it was wonderful. We had dinner at sunset at the Beach House, overlooking a blowhole, and on and on. Our wedding was the Saturday before Thanksgiving, so we could be gone nearly ten days and I would only need to be out of my office for three days.

We followed the same pattern for most of our yearly anniversaries. We'd go someplace fun over the Thanksgiving weekend, plus a couple of days. I don't remember where we went for the first few anniversaries, but on our fourth anniversary, we went to Santa Fe. I had tried to find a place where we could go skiing, but if there was no snow, we would still have something fun to do. We followed that pattern for about twenty years. Only about half the time were we able to ski, but we always had fun. We explored the galleries on Canyon Avenue, shopped at all the great shops around the Plaza, and had wonderful meals. Two of our favorites were Pasquals, a block off the Plaza, and Coyote Café. We stayed in various hotels, but our favorite was the St. Francis. They had high tea every afternoon in the lobby. I was disappointed when I visited Santa Fe a couple of years ago to see that they'd redone the lobby and gotten rid of the wonderful ambiance. It's now way too modern for me.

Alan and I were married for nearly twenty-five years, and it was wonderful, although we were opposites in many ways. I was very organized and precise—after all, I'm a lawyer. He was very creative and visionary. He was a Republican, I was a Democrat; he was conservative, I was liberal. He liked country music; I hated it. He was barely familiar with the Beatles; I was a big fan. I changed his mind on a lot of these things. He changed mine on others—like country music.

Nonetheless, we were compatible, too. We liked the same kinds of places to live; and had similar tastes in furniture, movies, food, and restaurants. We were both into yoga—in fact, several years later, he became an instructor. And we both loved traveling. We went to Europe several times and had a great time, and we also took lots of cruises. The first was through the Panama Canal, but we also went to Tahiti, Western Europe (England to Barcelona), and to the Caribbean several times.

We rarely fought. Alan often said that if you were struggling in your relationship, it wasn't working. We never struggled.

And we had a wonderful little dog, Pooh Bear, whom we both loved dearly. We'd gotten Pooh Bear when he was just a tiny puppy. I'm a dog lover, and I'd wanted one for years, but Alan wasn't quite so sure. Finally, I talked him into it. Pooh Bear was supposed to be a Maltipoo (half Maltese, half poodle), but as he grew, he looked less and less like one. He was bigger; with short legs, long silky white hair and a fluffy tail that curled over his back. We finally figured out that his litter must have had two fathers, and that he came from the second one.

He stuck with Alan and me like glue—unless he saw other dogs. He couldn't resist chasing them. One day he got out when we were both gone. Alan came home a little while later and was surprised to find Pooh sitting on the driveway, waiting for him in front of the garage.

Pooh also protected us. Alan worked at home, and I worked in an office and was gone all day. Usually, he ran out to greet me when I got home. But if Alan was taking a nap or not feeling well, he'd stay on the bed with

Alan and bark at me until I came into the bedroom, and then he'd roll over and wiggle until I rubbed his tummy.

Chapter 4

Alan's upbringing was very different from my middle-class one. His parents were musicians—not very successful ones. They'd moved from Indiana to Hollywood to make their mark, but they supported themselves with various low-wage jobs. His father managed a residential hotel for a while. I don't think his mother did much of anything. They were both alcoholics. His mother died when Alan was a senior in high school. She hadn't wanted Alan. Her child-rearing policy was that children should be seen and not heard. So, Alan stayed as quiet as he could and tried to disappear into the woodwork. He told me he'd sometimes had to steal food from the market when there was none at home.

His Aunt Jean became a second mother to him. She was only thirteen years older than he was, and she told him stories about her father, who'd been a successful businessman in Indiana—he owned a small phone company—until the Depression hit, and he lost everything. The main story Alan remembered was when his grandfather became enraged, hit his grandmother across the mouth with an umbrella, and knocked out all her teeth. Alan's grandfather, of course, did not approve of his daughter's choice of a husband and made life as miserable as he could for Alan's parents.

When Alan and I met, Aunt Jean was living in a funny little place in Henderson, Nevada—a town that had been built to house workers while they built Hoover Dam. We went and visited her often. After I'd been there several times, she told Alan that if he knew what was good for him, he'd marry me—immediately. It was, however, several years later before he got around to doing so. We were both heartbroken when she died of lung cancer a few years later. When Ronald and I moved to Vegas years later, we went looking for her house. I found the street, but wasn't sure about the house.

Alan was always a good student. When he graduated from Hollywood High School—in the same class as Carol Burnett—he went to the University of California at Berkeley to study engineering. But he joined a fraternity and had a little too much fun; he flunked out at the end of his freshman year and came back to LA, where he went to Los Angeles City College for a year until he was able to get his grades up. That was during the Korean War, so he joined the Marine Corps and went to Korea. He was a radar technician of some sort, so he didn't have to fight. But he told me about how dark it got at night where he was in Korea, and that the only way you could see someone passing while you were on guard duty was when the person blocked out the stars. They changed passwords every day, and if you didn't know the password, you'd be shot.

When Alan got out of the Marine Corps, he went back to Berkeley, buckled down, and graduated with a degree in electrical engineering. But because he'd flunked out in the beginning, he never thought he was very smart (my opinion was very different). He worked for various defense contractors all his career—sometimes in technical work, sometimes in sales, and sometimes on the management side.

When we met, he was working for the aerospace arm of TRW in Redondo Beach. By that time, he was a project manager managing work done by the company's subcontractors. Unlike a lot of technical people who can't make the transition from technical work to any kind of management, he did it very successfully.

Toward the end of his career, the defense industry was going through one of its periodic downturns, and the defense project he was working on was canceled. In an effort to keep many of its valuable employees, TRW started a study to use cutting-edge management technology to find a way to cut their costs in half— obviously, a very ambitious project. Alan was assigned to that project and spent a couple of years on it. They were successful in finding a way to cut costs in half, but when they were finished, they were unable to convince anyone in the company to adopt the new technology. They were all too entrenched in doing things the way they'd always done them. At that point, Alan was given the choice of taking early retirement or staying on at TRW and taking his chances with an eventual layoff. It didn't seem like much of a choice, so he took a not particularly generous early retirement package. We jokingly called it a brass handshake.

But Alan was still excited about the new management technology he'd been working on, so he tried to turn that into a management-consulting business. He worked with a couple of other guys who'd been laid off along with him on a program to use the new technology in consulting work. After a short time, the other guys went off in different directions, and Alan tried to go forward on his own. But he never found any paying clients—at least not any willing to pay a reasonable fee for his work.

He spent a lot of time working with my law school friend Mary Jo on a video she was developing on sexual harassment. It came out well, and she was able to market it to schools across the country for teacher training. We were living in Long Beach at that time, and Alan spent a lot of time on the road in his little red Miata, between Long Beach and Santa Barbara, where Mary Jo lived. Ultimately, he found it too difficult to work with a group of women—too much estrogen in the room, he said—but by that time, the project was done.

He also did a lot of work with our friend David in San Diego. David was trying to develop an integrated health-and-wellness center—similar to the kind you see all over the place these days—but he was never able to raise the necessary financing.

Chapter 5

I was born and raised in Pasadena, California. I had an older brother, Dick. He was fourteen when I was born and joined the Air Force when I was three, so I was essentially raised as an only child. I was around adults a lot, so I learned how to behave and not act like a kid.

I was always a "goody-two-shoes." I never caused any trouble for my parents, and I was never a rebellious teenager. Of course, things like drugs and alcohol were unheard of in the late '50s and early '60s when I was a teenager, and there was no social media or texting like there is for the kids today, so I had many fewer opportunities to get into trouble than kids do these days. And it was almost unheard of for girls to sleep with anyone while they were still in high school. My, how times have changed.

My mother was born in Wichita, Kansas, in 1907. Her family came to California when she was a teenager, with a one-year stop on a ranch in Arizona. She had four brothers, so her family provided me with lots of cousins while I was growing up. My father was born in Missoula,

Montana in 1909; his family moved to California when he was a kid. He had a sister, but she didn't have any children. Dad was a branch manager for Bank of America—he started in the mail room during the depression and worked his way up. My mother was a stay-at-home mom until I reached junior high school, when she went back to work as a legal secretary.

My mother was close to three of her brothers. The fourth (John) didn't speak to her after their mother died. My grandmother lived with us for the last few years of her life and I shared a bedroom with Nana. Because she provided a home, the agreement was that my mother didn't have to make any further financial contribution. The expenses were divided between the four boys. John's wife didn't think that arrangement was fair so she convinced him not to speak to my mother, or any of the other boys. That estrangement lasted until John divorced her when I was a teenager. He and my mother became quite close after that. She was visiting John and his second wife on the Big Island in Hawaii when she had a stroke and died in 1978.

I was closest to my mother as I was growing up. She was the one who guided me and influenced me. My father was a very sweet man, but he had no idea how to relate to a teenage girl. One night, when I as studying at the kitchen table after dinner, he came in and tried to strike up a conversation. Given my impatient streak, I imagine I wasn't particularly nice when I, in effect, told him to get lost. But my real bone of contention with him was his high opinion of my looks—too high, I thought. He was convinced that I would become the Rose Queen when I got to Pasadena City College (in those days, every girl at PCC was required to try out). Knowing that I could not fulfill my father's vision, I tried to avoid going there because I didn't want to disappoint him. But since that's where I went my freshman year, I had to do it. I didn't even make it past the first round of tryouts.

My father died of cancer about a year after my first marriage. The cancer had started as malignant polyps in his nose. He had them removed several times but, eventually, the cancer migrated into his brain. Things have really advanced since then and he would probably have lived a lot longer if the new treatments had been available. When I got married, he was sick enough that I had my brother on stand-by in case Daddy couldn't make it down the aisle. But he did make it. Several years later when my doctor said I had polyps in my nose that were causing my sinus headaches, I got really worried. But I had the surgery and there wasn't any problem.

My birthday is January 7. When I was growing up, I hated my birthday because it was so close to Christmas. Also, because it was in the winter, I couldn't have an outdoor birthday party in the park like all my friends. So, my mother, whose birthday was in July, and I negotiated to trade birthdays. Our negotiations broke down over the issue of which one of us was going to have to skip a birthday the first year.

My brother Dick joined the Air Force when he was seventeen and I was three. It was during the Korean War and he wanted to be a pilot. But it turned out he was color blind so he couldn't fly. But by then, he was stuck. He was based near Sacramento where he met a girl and married her when they were both nineteen. She already had a toddler and they soon had another one. Then they quickly had two more children, so I became an aunt when I was only five. His oldest child—Terry—is only five years younger than I am, so I grew up with his kids. Until I became an adult, Dick always seemed more like an uncle than a brother. My mother used to make Terry and me matching Easter dresses. I remember one year Terry's was pink organdy and mine was yellow.

When I was eight or ten, my brother and his family moved to Sacramento. I remember the road trips back and forth on Highway 99 to visit them. In those days, not only was the 99 only two lanes much of the way, but it went through the center of every small town between LA and Sacramento (and there are a lot of them). In those days, there was a big Bakersfield sign that straddled Highway 99. When they built a freeway through town, they refurbished the sign and moved it across a side street near Buck Owen's Crystal Palace.

My mother got pregnant again when I was four or five, but she had a miscarriage. Of course, at that age, I had no idea what a miscarriage was. For the longest time, my picture of a miscarriage was that when my mother went to the doctor, they took the baby out, put it on the counter, and shot it. How sick is that? I still remember the baby clothes that my mother had neatly laid out in dresser drawers in the spare bedroom.

Being raised in Pasadena, we almost always went to the Rose Parade, usually in the pre-parade area, where it was usually pretty chilly. My proudest moment was when I was about eight. I got a hug from Hopalong Cassidy! I'd watched him on TV at our next door neighbors (they got a TV before we did, so I used to go next door to watch the show with them). The younger brother in that household was a little terror. He was always chasing me around the back yard and biting me. My mother kept telling me to bite him back, but I wouldn't do it. One day when I ran crying to her, she took me back outside, caught hold of him, held his arm out and made me bite him. Guess she had the right idea. He never bothered me again.

When I was in fourth grade, we sold our house on the west side of Pasadena, rented a house in Eagle Rock for a year, then moved to the other end of Pasadena where my parents built a house in Sierra Madre (a small town at the northeast corner of Pasadena). From there, we were only about a mile from the end of the Rose Parade, so we'd often watch the entire Parade on TV, then walk down to the end and watch it go by again. I even stayed up all night on the parade route with my church group one year and sold roses in the morning to the crowd while we waited for the Parade to arrive. I was so sleepy when I got home that I fell asleep on the floor in front of the TV while the Rose Bowl game was on.

I went all the way through school in Pasadena. For kindergarten and the first three grades, I went to a school in my neighborhood where all the kids could walk to school together. I was only four-and-a-half when I started kindergarten. My mother often said she wished she'd held me back for another year, but all the kids in the neighborhood were starting school so she let me start with them. I developed slowly. I was in the slow reading group until I got to the third grade. Then I made it all up and moved all the way from the slow group to the first group in less than one school year. So ultimately, I think my mother made a good decision.

At the time, Pasadena had just gotten rid of what they called the 6-4-4 Plan—six years in elementary, four in junior high school, and 4 years in high school/junior college. The high school and junior college shared the same campus. They built a new high school (near where the Rose Parade ended) just in time for me to enter the 11th grade.

I was never particularly popular in high school—definitely not part of the "in crowd." I knew all of the popular girls, and they knew me—even years later when I'd see them at reunions. They were always nice to me. Coming mostly from wealthy homes, I was jealous of their clothes, particularly their Lanz dresses and angora sweaters. At that time, I was still making my own clothes at home.

I had my first real boyfriend was when I was a junior in high school. He turned sixteen while we were dating. His parents and friends threw him a surprise birthday party, but whoever was supposed to invite me dropped the ball. I got a frantic telephone call the afternoon of the party. Could I *please* come? We danced to *Sixteen Candles*—a popular song of the day. It was very romantic.

When that relationship petered out, I started dating one of his friends. David and I dated through the end of high school, then drifted apart when he went away to college in Berkeley. He and another friend drove me down to the ship when I went with my parents to Hawaii (in those days, they used to allow people on the ships, so we had a Bon Voyage party, champagne and everything).

There were several teachers who had a strong influence on my development in junior and senior high.

First was my social studies teacher in junior high who said he thought I should become an engineer. I thought he was crazy. After all, I hated math (even though I was always good at it). I didn't start liking math until I took algebra in high school where I took a machine-assisted class (just multiple choice tests that we graded ourselves). But it allowed us to move at our own speed. Even though I suddenly started to like math, I never thought any more about becoming an engineer and was later surprised when I found out that my chosen career at the time (architecture) required a lot of engineering courses.

Another teacher that influenced me at that time was my French teacher. My mother had made me take Spanish because so much of it is spoken in Southern California. Not a bad idea and I sometimes wish I'd stuck with it. But after two years of Spanish, I switched to French. The teacher was young, she'd lived in France for a while, and she made the language fun. I took two years in high school and another two in college, although the last year in college was a French Literature course. We had to read books by people like Sartre and Camus, in French. I would go to the library and get the book in English because the French was so hard. But even in

English, I still had trouble understanding them, philosophy never having been one of my strong suits. So I really struggled. It was the first time a teacher had ever sent home a deficiency notice to my parents. They were shocked and I was mortified. But I persevered and managed to bring my grade up to a C.

When I was in junior high, I also suffered from the cruelty of some teenage girls. Today, we would call it shunning. I was part of a group of four or five girls. We hosted parties together, had sleep overs, and generally did everything together. One of the girls had her class across the hall from mine right before lunch. We'd meet after class and go to lunch in the cafeteria together. One day, she wasn't there. I looked in her classroom. She wasn't there either. She'd simply abandoned me. She left me with no friends. At least that's what it felt like.

For a while, I was befriended by a couple of kids who were in what was considered the 'fast group' at school—not one I would have normally gravitated toward. But at the time, it felt like they'd saved my life. Gradually, I made other friends and never looked back. Years later, at a high school reunion, the friend who'd shunned me came up to me and wanted to know where I'd disappeared to way back then. I was shocked that her perception was so different from mine.

My social studies teacher my senior year in high school was probably the greatest influence of any teacher I ever had. He was of Japanese descent and had been born in Hawaii. The most upset I ever saw him was when some stupid boy asked him what Pearl Harbor had looked like from the air. He said he'd been eleven at the time.

Our term paper in that class was a really a lesson on how to write one (invaluable once I got to college). We picked our own topic and he taught us about research (we actually had to go to the library and look in books back in those days) and how to make notes on index cards, prepare an outline, and then arrange the cards in the right order based on the outline.

He also chose a group of us to make a photo project over Christmas Vacation (too early for video). We went down to the beach, in the December weather, in our bathing suits, and frolicked around in the sand. At least we didn't have to go in the water. When it was done, he showed it to all the home room classes—five or six times in one day. I gave a speech about the project at each of the sessions. One time, after having given the speech two or

50

three times, I froze. I can't remember how I got through that one.

His class was also where I discovered that I was smart. At some point, a rumor went around that you had to have an IQ of at least 120 to get into the class. I don't know if that was true, but it was definitely an advanced class. A friend of mine (who eventually became a doctor) was upset because he couldn't get into the class.

I graduated from Pasadena High School in 1962. My boyfriend my senior year went away to Cal Berkeley that fall and we wrote each other most every day, but it didn't last. It used to annoy him when I would complain about things that were happening in my life. I asked him who else I was supposed to talk to about things like that? When we broke up after the end of our freshman year, he said he hoped my next boyfriend would be more successful in getting into my pants. I was amused because he'd never even tried.

When I was eight or ten, I had a chance to impress everyone by getting to ride in the Queen for a Day Gold Cadillac. When we arrived at the theater where the popular show was filmed and climbed out of the car, everyone wanted to know who we were.

My Uncle Bob had created the show, and one day my mother, my sister-in-law and I met at his office and rode to the theater in the Gold Cadillac. Uncle Bob was my mother's older brother. As successful as he was, he'd never graduated from high school. When he was forty or fifty, he finally got his GED degree.

His son Robbie and I were very close growing up. He was about two years older than me. He had a sister, Marijoy, who was about two years older than my brother. Robbie was sent to a military academy for high school, then he joined the Navy. He married while he was in the Navy and had two kids. Their wedding reception was at his sister's lovely home in the Hollywood Hills. They received one wedding gift that mystified everyone. They finally had to ask what it was. It was a shallow oval silver dish with a curlicue attachment on one edge. Turns out it was for asparagus and the curlicue was supposed to hold the sauce. Who knew?

When Marijoy and her husband divorced a few years later, she got a degree in library science, moved to Eugene, Oregon, and became the college librarian at the

University of Oregon. Paul (my first husband) and I visited her there and enjoyed her lovely wood and glass home in a wooded area on the outskirts of Eugene. She had two daughters (I can't even remember their names). Eventually, she moved to Santa Rosa, California and became a librarian at one of the colleges there. My last contact with her was when Uncle Bob died in 1985. While she told me to please not come back from Europe for the funeral, I did see her some weeks later when she came down to close up his house. And a year or so later, she called me to ask if I could please call the probate attorney for Uncle Bob's estate to see if I could urge him, lawyer to lawyer, to hurry up and distribute the assets, which I gladly did.

Uncle Bob had a house high in the Hollywood Hills with a pool and a wonderful view of the surrounding hills—and the Hollywood Freeway. We always had a party by the pool on the 4th of July—fireworks and all.

My mother's younger brother, Jim, had two children. Jeff was about my age and his sister, Jean was a year or two younger. A second daughter was born several years later. Although Jeff and I were close, it was a long-distance relationship. One week during the summer, the two families met in Phoenix for a family vacation. We had great fun playing in the pool. But my Aunt Jane was one of those mothers who insisted that her kids eat every last bite on their plate before they could get up from the table. One day, Jean sat there for a couple of hours because she wouldn't finish her peas, while the rest of us were playing in the pool. I don't remember how that impasse ended, but eventually, it did.

Another summer, they all came to our house for a week. We had a ping pong table on the patio and we played so much ping pong while they were there that I had ping pong balls bouncing back and forth in my dreams.

Jeff and I graduated from high school the same year—1962. He went to Reed college in Oregon where he met a girl from Hawaii—she was half Chinese and half Portuguese. I think his parents disowned him—at least temporarily—when they married. Paul and I visited them in Honolulu for vacation shortly before I started law school. We got to experience Aloha Friday when all the men wore Aloha shirts to work; even my very proper cousin, who was an accountant. I think Aloha Friday was the precursor to Casual Friday, which is nearly universal now. We also went with them to a Friday-night party and watched a high school football game (high school football is probably almost as popular in Hawaii as it is in Texas). One of the players turned out to be one of the first Samoan players to make it in the NFL. My cousin's mother-in-law (the Chinese half) took us to dinner at a *real* Chinese restaurant with a big round table with a lazy susan in the middle. We had things I've never seen before, or since. It was a great vacation.

Unfortunately, I lost touch with Jeff and his wife not long after that. My mother was the one in the family who kept everyone together. After she died in 1978, I tried to keep in touch, but I never got much response. Eventually, I guess I just gave up. My Uncle Tom (another younger brother) died of a heart attack when he was only forty-two (which caused my mother to take driving lessons in case anything like that happened to her). Uncle Bob died in 1985 while Alan and I were in Europe. I last saw Uncle John when he was in a nursing home in Northern California (around 1980). Not sure what happened to him, although I assume he's long since dead.

I adored my Aunt Helen (Uncle Bob's wife). She was Swedish and I still see her making coffee her beautiful kitchen (even by today's standard) by putting the coffee grounds in a big coffee pot with an egg, shell and all. Of course, I was too young at the time to drink coffee, so I never got to taste it, but I understand now from Swedish friends that it's pretty good that way.

Aunt Helen always gave me wonderful Christmas gifts. One was a beautiful sequined sweater. I made a chiffon skirt to match it and wore it a lot for special occasions. I still have the sweater, although I haven't worn it in years. I just couldn't stand the thought of throwing it out. So this year, I bought some slinky gold pants and a matching tank top so I can wear it for things like New Years' Eve.

She also gave me a tiny gold heart on a chain. I wore it around my neck for years until I lost it when I was in college. I was sitting on a concrete bench in the middle of campus, between Dallas Hall and the Student Center, when I read my mother's letter telling me that Aunt Helen had died; I cried. About a month after she died, my heart broke again when I discovered I'd lost the little gold heart. Years later, after hearing me talk about it so much, Alan had a similar one made for me. I still wear it.

When I was in high school, I wanted to be an architect, but I discovered—a little late in the game—that it required a lot of science—the equivalent of a degree in civil engineering—and I wasn't up for it. But my mother was really against it. She couldn't see her fragile little girl competing in a man's world. At the time, it seemed like a pretty silly position—I was too young to understand things like discrimination against women, and the glass ceiling.

My second choice was fashion design. I had an artistic flair and I loved clothes. When I was little, I'd design and make clothes for my paper dolls and my Madame Alexander dolls. And I made all of my own clothes.

But for some reason, I didn't want to go to an art school. I wanted to get a liberal arts education at the same time. When I started checking out colleges when I was in high school, I could only find three that offered a major in fashion design—Rhode Island School of Design (RISDI), Syracuse University, and Southern Methodist University (SMU). Two things favored SMU. It was a lot closer to home, and it was much less expensive than the other two. Instead of the two years I would have been able to afford at Syracuse or RISDI, I could afford three years at SMU. So that's what I chose.

I went to Pasadena City College my freshman year and lived at home. I was essentially an art major—not a very good one. I took classes like life drawing (nudes) and design. We had some very unusual models in the life drawing class, but I found I liked them better than models with ordinary bodies—more curves and hollows. For years, I had three big pictures that I did in that class—one tissue paper collage and two charcoals. The collage is still hanging in a friend's home, but the two charcoal ones eventually fell apart.

I was a like fish out of water when I got to SMU. I'd never even visited the campus (not something college-bound kids did back in those days). Fortunately, my aunt and uncle had lived in Dallas some years earlier and they hooked me up with some friends of theirs who picked me up at the airport and dropped me off at my dorm. At that time, SMU was where the rich kids in Texas went if they couldn't get into an Ivy League School, or came back to when they flunked out of their fancy eastern schools. I knew nobody when I got there and had no idea how to meet people or make friends. Fortunately, the 'dorm' I was assigned to was a sorority house for a sorority that was starting a new chapter at SMU. There were fifteen or twenty other girls in the house and most of us became friends. I even ended up joining the sorority. My social life was handed to me without any further effort. It really helped.

Just like in high school, though, I was never really that popular while I was there. I never even had a boyfriend. I was engaged (secretly) to a guy back home named Scott. I met him on my summer job at Bullocks, but I dated at SMU anyway. The sorority was a help with women friends, but not so much when it came to guys. I went to some fraternity parties and had my share of blind dates, but nothing seemed to stick. I met one guy at a party (one of the ones who came back to SMU after flunking out of an Ivy League school) and dated him for several months, then he just seemed to evaporate. I met another guy in the library one night and dated him for several months. One night in the middle of winter, he walked me back from his apartment (after listening to the Beatles' Rubber Soul album, which had just come out). The streets were icy and I slipped and fell on my ass in the icy street.

The football game between Oklahoma University and the University of Texas was always at the Cotton Bowl in Dallas. It still is. And it was always a huge social event in Dallas. I usually had a blind date with some frat boy from Oklahoma, but nothing ever came of that either. One Saturday afternoon, some guy walked into my sorority house and yelled up the stairs—"does anybody want to go to a party?" He was an Army helicopter pilot based near Ft. Worth. I said yes and had several dates with him. I even visited him one weekend near the base. But then he was transferred somewhere else (the last stop before Vietnam) and I never heard from him again.

On Friday nights, a group of us who didn't have dates would go out to the home of one of my sorority sisters and her father, who was active politically in the Democratic Party, would regale us with tales of all his exploits while we ate popcorn and drank hot chocolate. Lots of fun, but not as good as a date. Their home was a big mansion (reminiscent of Mt. Vernon) overlooking the local lake.

And then there were the ordinary football games. SMU was not having a stellar period while I was there. Gone were the days of players like Doak Walker and

Dandy Don Meredith. While I was there, I saw Heisman Trophy winner Roger Staubach play for Navy (we won—one of the few football highlights while I was there). But the funniest thing came after SMU's game against Notre Dame the same year. In the days before the game, Ara Parseghian, the Notre Dame coach, was all over the local news saying that "wouldn't it be a hell of a note if the nation's number one football team went down to Dallas and got beat by a team that's not even good enough to be ranked?" Well, SMU didn't win the game. We only tied Notre Dame. When I got back to campus after the game, there was a banner on one of the sorority houses: "What a h... of a note!"

My senior year, the sorority planned a luau at the "Mt. Vernon" estate, but it rained for days during the preceding week. So, at the last minute, the mother made arrangements for us to have the luau at one of the downtown hotels—and she paid for it!

I had another blind date for the luau. He and I hit it off and we continued to date until the end of the school year. He wanted me to stay in Dallas after I graduated, but I wasn't that interested. When my parents came for my graduation, his father (who also would have liked me to stay after graduation) took us all out to dinner at the Petroleum Club at the top of one of the local skyscrapers. It was Memorial Day Weekend, so we were just about the only people in the place. The waiters were bending over backwards to take care of our table. His father had pre-ordered Beef Wellington for all of us. I had never even heard of it, but that didn't keep me from enjoying it. My parents were very impressed, which I'm sure was the idea behind all of it. But my parents weren't impressed enough to suggest that I stay in Dallas.

SMU was a very conservative school. Not so much because of the religious teachings, although we did have to take a year of religion—more like religious history than anything to do with dogma. We weren't allowed to wear slacks on campus and our curfew was pretty early relative to state schools. I was once chastised for wearing a mumu downstairs in the sorority house—someone called it a robe. And heaven forbid that there should be a co-ed dorm, or that boys would be allowed in your room. The world has certainly changed.

The student body —including me—was also very conservative. This was the middle of the Free Speech movement in Berkeley, and the height of the Vietnam

War, and anti-war protests were beginning around the country. But not at SMU. During my senior year, we were asked to sign a petition supporting the war, which I did. Our senior class president went with Bob Hope (or somebody like that) to deliver it to Vietnam. During my junior or senior year, the entire student body of the Divinity School took off for the south to help with voter registration. I was oblivious to all of it.

Even Religious Emphasis Week my senior year didn't make much of a difference. Each year, a prominent speaker would come to campus and spend a week speaking to us, giving seminars, etc. My senior year, it was the Rev. Sloane Coffin, from Yale. He set the campus on its ear with his speeches on discrimination. His point was that while fraternities and sororities might have the legal right to discriminate because of race or religion, they didn't have the moral or ethical right. I found it all quite interesting, but otherwise, I didn't pay much attention to it. However, one of my sorority sisters quit the sorority because of it. Some of the chapters had a lot of trouble with their particular universities when they wouldn't change their policy. Years later, I learned that the chapter at Wisconsin had to become independent so that it could stay on campus.

My consciousness didn't get raised until the antiwar movement reached its height during the 1968 primaries. That's also around the time I met Paul, whose family background in Massachusetts was blue collar Democratic. Once I got out of college, my views on race and the Vietnam War changed considerably. I was quite embarrassed some years later when I applied to become a bankruptcy judge. One of the questions on the application was whether you had ever belonged to an organization— private or not—that discriminated on the basis of race, sex, religion, etc. I had to say yes, and try to explain it away. Of course, my efforts to become a judge never went anywhere anyway, so my worrying was all for naught.

Also, we weren't allowed to leave Dallas without prior permission. One of the girls in the sorority house was dating a private pilot and they liked to rent an airplane and fly places on weekends. One weekend they invited me and another girl to fly with them to Oklahoma City, have dinner and fly back. All went well until it was time to return. There were thunderstorms in the area and we had to wait for a while to take off. That meant we had to call our housemother for "late permission" which would give us an extra hour beyond the normal curfew. But that also meant we had to call from a payphone without the operator saying anything that would let our housemother know we were in Oklahoma City. We talked to the operator and made sure she understood. It worked perfectly. I think it was after writing my mother to tell her of this latest adventure that she told me she wouldn't let my father read my letters until she had checked them first. That caught me totally by surprise.

The summer before I left for SMU, I went on vacation with my parents—we took the ship to Hawaii. We all had a really good time. The first day after we sailed, there were a couple of good looking guys sitting out on deck drinking beer. One of the men we'd met at our table at dinner said that his daughter and I should introduce ourselves, so we did. The four of us had a lot of fun for the rest of the trip, but when we got to Honolulu, we went one direction and the guys went another. We were gone for five days, then came back to Honolulu. My guy had left a message for me at one of the hotels we were staying at (at different times) and he was waiting for me when I got back. He'd extended his trip for a day so that we could spend more time together.

After we got home, we wrote each other fairly often and had occasional phone calls. After we both got to our respective colleges, I went to visit him at his home in Ohio for Thanksgiving (only days after the Kennedy assassination). I trudged through O'Hare Airport when I changed planes in Chicago. I'd checked as much luggage as was allowed (weight-wise) when I'd checked in for my flight in Dallas, but I was weighed down in Chicago by a train case and a bunch of books. I kept having to stop and rearrange things. Finally, I stuffed as many books as I could into the train case and checked it in Chicago. Worked like a charm.

In January or February the following year, I had an opportunity to drive to St. Louis with one of my sorority sisters (who'd gone to the same college as my boyfriend) and two other people who'd gone to Principia (near St. Louis) the year before. We all piled into the car and drove to St. Louis. It was an overnight trip so Sandy and I caught an early morning bus the next day and moved on to Jacksonville, Illinois. I had a great time with my boyfriend, but I nearly missed the return bus to St. Louis because I stayed to watch the Beatles in their first appearance on the Ed Sullivan Show. At that point, I had no idea who the Beatles were (I was kind of slow when it came to things like that). Once I got back to campus, my boyfriend and I just kind of drifted apart.

My senior year, my twenty-first birthday fell during first semester finals. My roommate tried to commit suicide that evening. I found her in the maid's room. She'd taken a bunch of sleeping pills. I was horrified. Fortunately, she didn't succeed. We were very close. Then, after that tragic event, when I tried to find someone who was willing to buy me a drink to celebrate, the only person I could find was another of my close friends who was not yet twenty-one herself. So, we went to the same bar that never asked for ID anyway, and she did bought me a beer.

After her suicide attempt, my roommate was taken off to some mental hospital. After a few weeks, her parents came from Maryland and took her home. I didn't see her again until our first sorority pledge class reunion ten or fifteen years later. She shared with us her experiences at the mental hospital—being raped with a broomstick handle and things like that. Because she'd never heard from any of us after she went home, she thought we knew what had happened and didn't care. I was heartbroken when I heard her story. I'm so glad she came to the reunion and we were able to tell her how much we all loved her. She died a few years later (she'd always had horrible health problems).

We've had several more sorority pledge class reunions, but I've only made it to one. It was at a working ranch outside Dallas that was owned by the family of one of the members. The ranch was used for corporate retreats so it had lots of luxury accommodations—a lot like a small resort hotel (without the pool or other resort amenities). The reunion was well-planned, with the local members planning all the menus and doing all the grocery shopping. We all shared in the cooking and clean-up, and each of us planned a particular segment of the meeting— mine was photo memories—everyone brought their family photos that covered the years since we had graduated. There's been one more reunion and while I had great intentions of going, it ended up being only a week or two before my wedding on Halloween in 2010, so I didn't go. We've exchanged lots of emails since then, but with our advancing ages, I doubt that we'll ever get together again.

Chapter 6

There were a lot of reasons why SMU turned out to be a poor choice for college. First, at the end of my junior year, SMU discontinued the fashion design program, which meant that I had to cram all the courses for my major in before the end of my junior year, leaving me with only academic courses for my senior year—a bit tough.

One of the academic courses that I took that year was abnormal phycology. I was dating a guy who was a psych major and he offered to let me use his abnormal psych term paper, which he'd gotten an A on. It was on existential psychology; I didn't even know what that meant. So, I decided that I couldn't just re-write it without understanding what I was I was saying. I researched it from scratch to the point that I almost understood what I was saying. I got a B. My parents came to Dallas for my graduation at the end of that year. The day they arrived, I'd just gotten the postcard with my final grade in the mail. When my parents pulled up in front of the sorority house, I went running out to greet them, waving my grade card in the air and shouting "I got an A in Abnormal." My father's response was, "This is what I sent you to college for?"

The other academic course that gave me trouble was Biology. I'd taken it in high school and hadn't had a problem. I also had to take a course in chemistry or physics in order to graduate, so I took chemistry my junior year. I was scared to death of it so I really studied, making sure that I knew the entire table of chemical elements, backwards and forwards. I got 100 on the first test and an A for the first semester. But at the end of my first semester of biology, I got a D. I think it was a combination of the biology lab (we hadn't had lab in high school) and my inability to recognize the slides on the test, along with the fact that biology lab was my only 8 a.m. class that semester. I did so poorly that I was worried I wouldn't make a D for the final semester (I needed at least a D in order to graduate). I think I got a C.

With the fashion design program having terminated at the end of my junior year, I also had no support from the placement office when it came time to find a job. So, I moved back home to Pasadena. By then, my parents had sold our house in Sierra Madre and were moving to a condo in Torrance with a nine-hole pitch and putt golf course. They took me down and showed me the models. When we went out on the second floor balcony of the model, you could see an oil derrick in the parking lot and I said, "boy, I wouldn't want to be in this location." My parents said that the unit they were buying was right downstairs. Oops!

I lived in Pasadena after I graduated. A year later, I moved into an apartment in Torrance and visited my parents often. I even played golf with them on their golf course. Of course, I thought that was pretty nifty until a guy I was dating invited me to play with him on a full-length course. That may have been the last time I played golf. I really embarrassed myself.

But I didn't find out until after I graduated how bad my choice of SMU had really been. I could have gone to a school like RISDI and gotten a good education in both design and liberal arts (by taking academic courses at Brown). Or I could have gone to a liberal arts college and then to art school for a master's in fine arts. But there was nobody around to give me that kind of advice. My high school guidance counselor didn't know any more than I did about becoming a fashion designer.

When I graduated from SMU, I came back home to Pasadena and shared an apartment with a friend from high school. She'd been married briefly and had a two-year-old daughter. That was quite an adventure.

After a short search, I got a job with a small sportswear manufacturer (they made clothes for Penny's) as an assistant patternmaker. But after an eight-week probation period, I was let go. That's when I found out just how lacking my education at SMU had been. My fashion design career didn't survive.

But I had to figure out what I was going to do to earn a living because living at home wasn't an option. My father put me in touch with someone in personnel at Bank of America, and I became a teller at the Los Angeles Main Office. Not exactly my idea of a brilliant career. I was there for a couple of years and got one promotion—to foreign exchange teller. It was during the Vietnam War and a lot of my work was sending money from paychecks to construction workers in Vietnam (a job that I'm sure is done now with the punch of a button on a computer). But I also got another chance to use my Spanish. By the time

I was done, I could cash a check or sell a money order in Spanish.

But after a couple of years, I quit and looked for a secretarial job, hoping I could find one in a more interesting business. I got a fortuitous break—one of many in my life. I was hired as a secretary in the media department (the people who figure out where to spend the advertising dollars) of an ad agency, which I enjoyed very much. I had several jobs in advertising, then settled at a small agency in Century City.

During that time, I met and married Paul. We met in the TV room of the South Bay Club in Torrance—the original "swinging singles" apartment complex—where we both lived, and started dating. I'd moved into the apartment about a year after I got out of college. It was the first time I'd ever found myself really popular with guys. I never lacked for a date and I thoroughly enjoyed myself for the better part of a year. And then I met Paul.

We dated exclusively for some months until he proposed, keeping it secret for several months. We bought a ring and made it official at Christmas. We got married in June 1969 in the Catholic Church.

The most memorable moment of the wedding was when my maid of honor fainted! When I started back up the aisle, I was surprised that it was the deacon (a man, of course) who handed me my bouquet. But when I got to the other end of the aisle and turned around, there she was behind me. She was positively green.

The second best moment was when we got the wedding pictures back. The photographer caught my flower girl, Kimberly, with her finger in the frosting of the wedding cake. When Kimberly saw the picture, she told her mother, "Mommy, I didn't touch it!" The evidence to the contrary, however, was right in front of us.

I stayed in advertising for four or five years—until I started law school—and was eventually promoted to media buyer. But it still wasn't the career I'd hoped to find, so I started thinking about going back to school. I wanted an education that would actually qualify me for a career (unlike my college degree, which hadn't qualified me for much of anything). My first thought was to get an MBA so that I could become an account executive in advertising.

I took the entrance exam and was ready to start applying to local graduate business schools when I had an epiphany: why not go to law school instead? It sounded much more interesting. A friend of mine had just finished law school, and she'd loved it. I ran the idea by my husband, Paul, but he didn't think it was such a great idea. When he came around a week or two later, I realized that I'd made the decision so quickly (a Capricorn trait) that he didn't think I really knew what I was doing. My mother, on the other hand, had made a 180-degree switch from her earlier attitude about my working in a man's world, and thought it was a great idea. She'd been a legal secretary most of her life and had once been urged to go to law school herself. She couldn't have been more supportive. I guess it shows what eight years and a women's movement can do.

I took the LSAT—the entrance exam for law school—and did very well. I started applying. Unfortunately, there'd been a lot of grade inflation during the eight years since I'd graduated from college, so even with my really good LSAT scores, it wasn't easy to get into a good law school. My first choice was UCLA, which was ranked very well nationally and was close to home. I made the waiting list but never got in. My next choice was Loyola University School of Law, also in Los Angeles. Because I was married, and Paul had a good job in the LA area, I never applied to any of the better law schools anywhere else. I've often wondered if I could have gotten in.

I'd been warned that the studying process in law school is a lot different from the kind I was used to in college, and that the results wouldn't necessarily be the same. So, I determined how many hours a week I was willing to study, and decided that I would be satisfied, whatever the outcome. Apparently, I hit the mark, because I did very well. At the end of my first year, I was second or third in my class, and by the time I graduated, I was number three in the daytime class, and number five when combined with the night class. Not too bad. I was definitely satisfied with that result.

Chapter 7

But then came the job hunt. Graduating fifth in my class should have guaranteed a lot of good job offers, even though Loyola wasn't a first tier law school; not even in LA. Not so for me. For the summer after my second year, I interviewed with a number of top Los Angeles firms but never even got a callback. When school was almost out for the year, one of my friends from Law Review said he could get me an interview at the firm he would be working when he graduated—McKenna & Fitting, a good midsize firm in LA. I jumped at the opportunity and spent the summer working there with about eight other summer clerks.

At that time, if you did well during the summer, you would be offered a permanent job at the end of law school. Actually, you had to be pretty bad not to get an offer, so I was shocked when I didn't receive one. The reason they gave me was that my writing wasn't very good. Even then, I knew that was bullshit. After all, you can be taught to write, can't you? So, I moved on, not knowing the real reason.

But because of what that firm said, I've always paid a lot of attention to my writing style over the years, even taking several classes in legal writing. The best lesson I ever had, however, was one day a few years later when I was working at a good bankruptcy firm. I gave one of the partners a draft of something I'd written, and he went through it and marked it up. When he was done, he pointed to one spot where he'd put a red question mark. He said that I'd eventually gotten around to answering his question later in the brief, but the place where he'd put the question mark was where the answer should have been. I've always remembered that lesson and tried to make sure I put my facts and arguments in the best order. After all, that's what legal writing is all about—argument and persuasion.

Years later, I finally figured out what I now think was the real reason why I didn't get an offer that summer. When I got out of law school, firms had barely started hiring women (in spite of the fact that my law school class was about a third women); and I think they figured that having hired one or two women, that was all they needed to do. How wrong they were. These days, slightly more than half of law school graduates are women, and the number of job offers is about the same. But women still have trouble breaking through the glass ceiling to partnership.

For my last year of law school, I had a lot of free time (many law students think the entire third year is a waste of time), so I got a part-time job at a small entertainment firm in Century City. And while I went through the whole interview process with the big firms again, the result was the same—zip, zilch, nada. So, when the firm I was working for part-time offered me a permanent job, I took it, even though the salary was pretty pathetic.

I stayed there for about a year working on small cases, family law, et cetera. But one day as I was preparing a case for trial, I realized that a significant piece of evidence was missing. When I talked to the partner in charge of the case, his solution was to create a paper trail and backdate it. That didn't sit well with my ethical streak, so I talked with a different partner about what had happened, told him that I was quitting because of it, and said that I expected him not to oppose my unemployment claim. He agreed. I have no idea what he did after that about the fraudulent evidence.

Meanwhile, I started looking for a new job. A friend from law school told me about a job that was opening up at Getty Oil Company and suggested I apply. At that time, the idea of working for an oil company was not something that particularly appealed to me (my liberal streak had long-since revealed itself). But my friend said that his friend had told him it really wasn't so bad. I applied and got the job. It involved working with the price regulations that controlled gasoline prices at the time. I knew nothing about the field, but neither did many other people. Plus, as a second-year lawyer, nobody expected me to know that much. It was interesting and challenging. It was only a few months later when I met Ronald at a seminar in Houston, and my life has never been the same.

I had fun at that job. I got to travel a lot, to Tulsa, Philadelphia, Washington, San Francisco and other places. I was on an expense account, so I always stayed in nice hotels and ate at good restaurants. The Thanksgiving after Ronald walked out, I spent several days in San Francisco at that beginning of that week with our outside litigation firm, and then drove to my brother's in Sacramento. At least, that was the idea. I left around noon on Wednesday, intending to cross the Bay Bridge to the east side of the Bay and continue on from there. Unfortunately, there'd been a chemical spill earlier that day near the access to the bridge and the whole thing was closed. I did the only other thing I knew to do—I crossed the Golden Gate Bridge into Marin County and took the Richmond Bridge across to the east side of the Bay. With everyone else doing the same thing, the traffic was, as you can imagine, a nightmare. I stopped at least twice to call my sister-in-law who was waiting for me at her office in Sacramento. As it got later and later, I finally told her to go home and I would go directly to their place. Once I finally got there, I had a really nice visit. Somewhere along the line, I took my rental car into Sacramento and turned it in. On Sunday, we all drove to San Francisco for a Forty Niners game against the LA Rams. After the game, my brother dropped me off at my hotel in SF and drove back to Sacramento.

The main focus of my job at Getty was to determine what Getty, and its affiliate Skelly (in Tulsa), had charged for a gallon of gas during the first Arab oil embargo a few years earlier. The permissible price in 1979—the second oil embargo—started with the price on the target date, adjusted upward or downward for various changes that had occurred in the meantime. Because the oil companies hadn't been able to raise prices enough after the end of the first embargo to come anywhere near the cap, they hadn't bothered to keep very good records of the price cap, or the changes in service that had occurred in the intervening years. My job was to go around to the various offices, work with the accounting department, and try to figure out the base price, and based on that, the permitted current maximum price at that time. Not an easy job. The other half of my job was to provide litigation support to the outside law firm in San Francisco that handled the company's litigation against the Department of Energy (DOE). It was that part of the job that took me to San Francisco that Thanksgiving.

After a couple of years, however, some major changes occurred that quickly ended my career in the regulatory field. First, Getty entered into a global settlement with the DOE that ended all the litigation I was working on (about half my workload). I asked the head of the legal department to give me something else to do, but my request fell on deaf ears. This was shortly before Ronald Reagan was elected president in 1980, and the writing was already on the wall, so I quit Getty. Once

Reagan was elected, of course, the price regulations were quickly taken off the books, as we'd all expected, and my job would have died along with it.

I took three or four months off to play in politics. I worked on John Anderson's third-party presidential campaign. My first political campaign was eight years earlier when George McGovern was the Democratic nominee. The advertising agency I worked for at that time handled McGovern's California primary campaign and I was the media buyer assigned to handle the account. A political campaign is a different breed of cat from any normal ad campaign. First, it's a huge project in a short amount of time. It was fast and furious for the eight weeks or so that the campaign lasted. At one time or another, most us were looking for some Valium to handle the stress. We hired several freelance buyers to help. And then there's the media buys themselves. At that time, the media had to sell political advertising at the lowest cost they'd sold anything in the last year to any other advertiser. We had to keep extremely good records of the advertising we purchased because we would be—and were—audited after the campaign.

We worked closely with the local McGovern campaign staff. At one meeting, the black campaign staff was whining about the attention that the Hispanic group was getting because Hispanics generally failed to get out the vote the way the blacks did. From what I read about this year's campaign, that part hasn't changed.

But the funniest thing that happened during the campaign was the phone call I got one day from my niece, Terry. She was at the Democratic Convention and they were looking for one of the TV ads that had run in California and someone told her I was the person to call. We still laugh about that one.

For the last month or two of the 1980 Anderson campaign, I drove what had become known as the "death car"—the car in a motorcade that's right behind the Secret Service van with all the guns. The death car carries the pool reporters. The van's job was to defend the candidate in case of attack. Of course, there was no attack, but we tried to spice things up a bit by renting fun cars. Most often, it would be a vintage Cadillac convertible, big as a boat. While the event was taking place inside, I hung out with the reporters. Driving in a Motorcade was its own adventure, but it was fun. Sometimes, because it was a third-party candidate, we didn't even have a police escort to stop traffic. We were on our own.

In the meantime, however, I needed some income. When I couldn't find a job in the regulatory field (not surprising, since nobody was hiring), I took a part-time job with a small firm in West LA doing hourly work on various litigation matters. And then a new career opportunity opened up. One of the lawyers affiliated with the firm—Dick—was a bankruptcy attorney, and I started learning bankruptcy law by working with him. One day when I called someone to get information on a case for him, they asked me if it was a Chapter 7 or a Chapter 11. I didn't even know the difference, but I learned quickly.

After a few or months of contract work, I opened my own office, renting a small space in the same building. There were three or four other attorneys in the suite. I had no secretary, but I shared the receptionist and the copy machine. I bought my first computer from Radio Shack— the kind where you had to insert a floppy disk with the software, then take that floppy out and insert another one in order to save anything. The scariest thing that happened during those days was when my computer ate the directory on one of my floppy disks so I couldn't access anything that was saved on the disk. Fortunately, I'd printed out almost all my documents. I only had to reinvent one of them. I think this was around 1980. I'm sure glad that times have changed, although I have had my issues with computers crashing and the like.

Being a boss, I was amazed to learn how much kids—even middle class kids—didn't learn at home when they were growing up. I hired a high school student to help out in the office. Among other things, he was responsible for the outgoing mail. One day he told me that we were out of stamps. I was flabbergasted. Didn't it occur to him that we needed to buy more stamps *before* we ran out?

During that time, I got a lot of my work from my mentor, Dick. He represented one of the local bankruptcy trustees and did most of that trustee's real estate work. I learned from him as I went along. I also learned bankruptcy by working part-time at a legal clinic in Whitter—a forty-five-minute drive from my West LA office. The clinic filed a lot of Chapter 7 cases for individuals without any nonexempt assets—known in the trade as "no asset cases." The clinic brought in an outside bankruptcy attorney, and he gave me a one-day seminar on Chapter 7s. I was off and running. Once I felt comfortable handling them, I started to advertise for my own Chapter 7 cases. People often ask how you get paid by people who are filing bankruptcy. Easy. You charge a flat fee, and you make sure it's paid up front.

I continued building my own practice for the next several years. I even started handling small Chapter 11 business cases. But as my practice grew, so did my overhead. After five years or so, while my gross income had gone up a lot each year, my net income wasn't any more than I had made in the beginning. And that wasn't very much. I was going further and further into debt, living off credit cards and a line of credit from my lawyer-friendly bank. Finally, I realized I was going nowhere.

One day several years before I had this come-to-Jesus talk with myself, Ronald had called me about handling a major litigation matter for Oxy, where he was still working. It killed me to refer it to my friend Mary Jo, but as a sole practitioner, I simply couldn't handle anything that big. Her firm put four or five lawyers on the case, and they worked around the clock for several days getting the lawsuit ready to file. But that was the kind of legal work I wanted to handle. The disappointment of not being able to handle that case had festered for several years.

Finally, I realized I was spending as much time on my practice's administrative matters—I was sharing an office and a secretary with Dick—as I was doing work that generated fees. So, after much thought and discussion with Alan (we'd gotten married a couple of years earlier), I decided to close my office and look for a job. A friend referred me to a headhunter who specialized in placing bankruptcy attorneys, and he found me a *very* good job— the kind I had no reason to think I was even qualified for.

Gendel, Raskoff, Shapiro & Quittner was one of the best bankruptcy firms in the Los Angeles area. All the named partners were considered "deans of the bankruptcy bar"—not just locally, but nationally. Of course, the current bankruptcy law was still pretty much in its infancy at the time. The prior Bankruptcy Act had been thrown out in 1978 and replaced by the Bankruptcy Code. So in 1988, the law was still developing. Gendel Raskoff hired me as a senior associate, with a salary to match (about four times what I'd been taking home as a sole practitioner). I think they sometimes wondered if I knew as much as they expected me to. At the time, I was pretty good at what I knew, but there were a lot of issues I'd never handled and therefore didn't know much about. But what did they expect? I'd never even taken a course in bankruptcy law when I was in law school, and I'd been a sole practitioner with a very limited client base. The firm's second thoughts also fueled my innate fear that people might discover that, underneath my façade as a successful lawyer, I was really stupid.

But I was a quick learner, and after a couple of years, I think everyone was happy with my work. By the time the firm dissolved in 1993, I'd gotten the highest bonus among the associates, and I was ready for partnership. Too bad my timing was off.

About two years after I was hired, the firm took on a huge Chapter 11 business case in St. Louis. We thought we were being hired as special counsel to help out the small St. Louis firm that had filed the case. The senior partner told me I'd need to travel to St. Louis once or twice a month for two or three days at a time. But by the time three of us attorneys flew to St. Louis one afternoon and met at the local attorneys' offices the next morning, we were the *only* firm handling the case. The prior afternoon, while we were on the plane, the judge had disqualified the firm from further representation of the company based on some conflicts of interest. And by the time that happened, every other bankruptcy attorney in St. Louis was already representing someone else in the case.

Boy, did that change things. Instead of once or twice a month, I started spending the better part of three weeks a month in St. Louis. It was very hard on Alan. While I almost always made it home on weekends, I was usually gone for four or five days a week. He turned to friends when it got especially hard, but I was finally working on the kind of complex case that I'd always wanted to work on.

At the time, Apex Oil Company was probably the largest private company ever to file for Chapter 11 bankruptcy protection. These days, of course, it's become a fairly common business strategy used by huge corporations. The stigma is gone.

This traveling went on for the better part of three years, but Alan and I did get to do some fun things while it was going on. I accumulated a lot of airline miles on TWA, which we used for several nice vacations, all first class. We went once or twice to Europe and once to the Caribbean. And Alan periodically visited one of his clients in New Jersey, so a couple of times when I was in New York at the same time, we were able to rendezvous in Manhattan for dinner. One weekend, we stayed in the company brownstone not far from Bloomingdale's. I showed him how to get around on the subway—a talent that I found doesn't take that long to acquire. But first, I had to convince him that renting a car at the Newark Airport and driving into Manhattan would not be a good idea. While he was there, we had brunch at Tavern on the Green and went dancing at the Rainbow Room. And, of course, we shopped at Bloomingdale's. Also, the NY office gave us a couple of tickets to a Knicks game at Madison Square Garden. Then, on Monday, Alan went off to his work in New Jersey, and I flew home.

Once Gendel Raskoff realized it was on its own with the St. Louis case, we opened a St. Louis office and staffed it with a couple of local attorneys (the firm that had originally handled the case imploded after it was disqualified, so we hired two of its lawyers). So, it was easy for us to do our work while we were there. Although the LA attorneys who were working the case weren't licensed to practice in Missouri, it was Federal Court, and the judge handling the case didn't seem to mind if we appeared without local counsel being with us (not the same as in LA), so we handled all the court appearances pretty much by ourselves. Sometimes there would be four or five of us handling different court matters on the same day.

Although being away from home so much was rough—on me as well as on Alan—I also learned a lot about handling a complex business case. I worked late most nights while I was in St. Louis so that I could take the weekends off when I was at home. Whatever attorneys were in St. Louis at the time often had dinner together at various local restaurants. There were usually four to six of us. We were on an expense account, so we ate well, went to all the best restaurants, and consumed a fair amount of good wine. Interestingly, the Bankruptcy Court—which had to approve our fees—never objected to those expenses. I think the only expense that was ever denied was somebody's in-room movie rental. The other restriction the judge put on us was the travel time. He would only allow us to bill for two hours on the airplane (the estimated time to travel from Chicago to St. Louis). The rest of the time, we tried to do billable work on the plane so that we could get paid.

The case finally ended and, before long, I was out of a job when Gendel, Raskoff fell apart. It wasn't unusual at that time for firms to go under for financial reasons. But not Gendel Raskoff. It went under because the partners couldn't agree on a future direction for the firm. Stupidest thing I've ever seen. One year the partners would decide they wanted to develop a full-service practice by adding corporate, securities, real estate, and so on, and the partners that wanted it to stay as a small boutique firm would leave. Then the next year, the partners would decide to remain as a boutique bankruptcy practice and the partners that wanted to go full-service would leave. Finally, they voted to seek a merger with a full-practice firm. But by that time, however, the firm no longer had the critical mass necessary to survive as an independent firm of any size.

For the better part of a year, the firm negotiated with various national firms. The firms all wanted our bankruptcy practice, but Gendel refused to let anybody cherry-pick among our attorneys. They had to take the whole package. After getting close a couple of times, there was no merger. I was devastated. I'd finally found my dream job, and now it was being snatched away from me. Some years later, one of the senior partners asked me what I thought had happened. I said I didn't know, but all the time I was thinking, *if you don't know, how do you expect me to?*

Not long before the end, a group of attorneys left and opened a local office for a small San Francisco bankruptcy firm. Another group joined a large litigation firm in downtown LA. And a third group went to the LA office of a New York firm—Stroock & Stroock & Lavan. I was part of the third group (I'd interviewed for a lot of other jobs but hadn't gotten any offers).

I hated Stroock from the day I got there. The LA office was nothing but a poor stepchild to the New York office. Only one of our bankruptcy attorneys was ever given a chance to work on a New York case. The rest of us had no interaction with any of the New York bankruptcy attorneys. I never even met any of them.

In addition, the bankruptcy department was understaffed and overworked (an oxymoron?). I quit working such long hours once I realized that no matter how hard I tried, I couldn't keep up with my cases. I focused only on the most urgent matters. The problem was exacerbated by the fact that the firm's reputation as a place to work was so bad that we couldn't even hire anybody.

And I didn't particularly like the attorneys I was working with. A classic example was when one partner sat me down to chew me out over a management decision I'd made. First off, of course, management decisions were not part of my job. I'd just been trying to get something done that needed quick attention while my boss was out of town. When I tried to defend my handling of the matter, he looked at me and said, "Well, sweetie . . ." in a very demeaning tone. There was another partner in the office at the time. We looked at each other, and I could tell he'd thought the comment was as offensive as I had. I didn't say another word. I just picked up my papers and left the room. Eventually, after I'd talked to one of the other partners, I got a halfhearted apology.

I also had another problem while I was there. I went with one of the partners I'd worked with for years at Gendel, Raskoff up to Santa Barbara to pitch a new client. We planned to stay overnight with some of his friends. It never occurred to me to ask if the friends would be there. I just assumed they would. I didn't find out until I got there that they weren't going to be home. But I didn't think too much about it at the time. After all, I'd worked with this man for years and considered him to be both a mentor and a friend. Silly me. When we got to the house after dinner, he tried to kiss me. I said no, and he backed off, but it certainly made for a sleepless night.

This all happened while the Clarence Thomas/Anita Hill Supreme Court confirmation hearings were going on, and we were all learning a lot about sexual harassment, including the need to immediately tell somebody what had happened. So, when I got home, I told Alan, as well as a friend who was visiting. The partner and I resumed our working relationship without another word being spoken. But it certainly woke me up.

Somewhere around that time, I decided that even if Stroock was to offer me a partnership, I didn't want to be partners with any of their attorneys, so I started looking for another job. I went back to the same headhunter I'd used before, and I was hired by Jeffer, Mangels, Butler & Marmaro, a top-notch, medium-size firm headquartered in Los Angeles. I did well, and I enjoyed the work. Management, however, was another story. The managing partner was a stern taskmaster, seemingly more concerned with making money than with the quality of the legal product, although the work produced by the firm still somehow managed to be very good.

But I had several run-ins with management over money. The bigger bankruptcy cases sometimes don't pay their lawyers until the end of the case because the court has to approve the payment of legal fees. And, once in a while, if the business ultimately fails, they don't get paid at all. I had a couple of cases that ended up in the latter category.

At one point, I was working on a case for a major bank client. After a year or so of litigation that seemed to be going nowhere, the bank put a limit on the fees it would pay for the rest of the case, and the limit was pretty low given the discovery work we were in the middle of. While I was vaguely aware of the limit, and the fact that we would soon blow through it, I had two partners above me on the case, and I expected them to deal with management on the issue and either get the limit raised or tell me to quit working. Silly me. They did neither, and I was left holding the bag. I was fired.

Chapter 8

By the time I was fired, Alan and I had been wanting to get out of Los Angeles for several years. We decided this was our chance. The question was where to go. We started with a trip to Bend, Oregon, to check it out. I had a friend there—a paralegal I'd worked with at Stroock. She was doing exactly what I wanted to do— working long-distance from home. She showed us around and introduced us to a real estate broker friend of hers. Homes were unbelievably cheap, and we loved Bend, but we weren't through exploring our options.

Our next trip started in Durango, Colorado. Like Bend, I knew someone who knew someone, who introduced us to his real estate agent. We liked the town, and the prices were right. From there, we drove to Taos, New Mexico. We'd planned on staying for three or four days, and we'd hoped to ski (it was around Thanksgiving), but there was no snow. We didn't care for Taos as a place to live (way too small), and when we couldn't find anything much else to do there, we drove down to Santa Fe (about an hour away).

We'd spent a lot of time in Santa Fe over the years and loved it. But we didn't think we could afford it. The big surprise was that if we didn't try to buy something in the middle of town, it was surprisingly reasonable. By the time we got home, we'd decided to move to Santa Fe. We even made a couple of trips back there to look at homes and made an offer on one, but somebody else got there first.

But we weren't going anywhere until we sold our place in Long Beach. We'd found it while I was looking for a job right before Gendel shut down. I had a couple of job possibilities in Orange County, so we went down to the Long Beach area, thinking it might be a good place to live, halfway between Orange County and Alan's job in Redondo Beach.

While we were wandering around, we spotted some great-looking new houses across the water on a marina. The development was called Spinnaker Bay, and a lot of the houses came with their own boat slips. Alan loved sailing, so he was sold.

They were pretty expensive, compared to where we were living, but they were really nice. Plus, of course, we were both employed and had a pretty good income. We bought the smallest model; one that had fallen out of escrow, so the asking price was a bit on the low side. We placed our condo on the market and it sold immediately.

Not only was the new house a lot bigger and nicer than where we'd been living, but it came with a boat slip. Once we moved in, we started looking for a sailboat. We bought a Cal 20 from a woman who was planning to give it to charity. It was old and didn't look very good, but it was fundamentally sound. She sold it to us for $500—the amount she figured her charitable deduction was actually worth to her. We put about $1,000 into fixing it up, including some rigging that allowed us to lower the mast so we could get under the Second Street Bridge and out to the ocean. Then we started enjoying it.

I'd never done much sailing, so Alan taught me to sail. I loved it and became an active member of our two-person crew. We also enjoyed taking friends and family out sailing. Living on Alamitos Bay, it took us about twenty minutes to motor out to the ocean. We went out almost every weekend. With the boat right outside our back door, we could decide to go sailing and be under way in about fifteen minutes, picnic lunch and all.

We also bought a small electric boat that we used to motor around the bay and through the canals of Naples Island. It was great for entertaining, and we could even motor to some of the local restaurants. During the summer, there were outdoor concerts at one end of the nearby Marine Stadium (where they held the rowing events during the 1932 Olympics). We'd pack a picnic dinner and join lots of other boats anchored nearby. Then we'd motor home. Of course, the electric boat had no toilet, which made the return trip a bit challenging on a couple of occasions.

But once our first grandchild was born, we had to choose between sailing and visiting with the baby. The baby usually won.

We'd no sooner moved into the Long Beach house than Alan took early retirement, so we were without his salary. A few years later, when I lost my job, we had *no* regular income. Alan had tried to start a consulting business, but he never got that off the ground. I worked from home and was a bit more successful in the income department, but mine was pretty sporadic, and our house payments were nearly $3,000 a month, so it was a bit stressful. I don't think Alan ever forgave me for deciding to sell the Long Beach house, but at the time, there was really no choice.

We spent about nine months getting the place ready to list—why it took us so long, I have no idea. Then we listed it. It was a really bad real estate market, so it sat on the market for another nine months without one offer.

One day Alan asked me if my plan to telecommute was really going to work if we moved to Santa Fe. I had to say no. Law firms just weren't ready for it yet. So what did that mean? We decided the only thing that made sense was to move back up to the West LA area where most of my free-lance legal work was coming from. About two weeks later, we got our first offer on the house. Although it was substantially less than we'd paid for the place, it was fairly reasonable, given the weak market at the time. After some negotiation, we accepted it and started looking for a place in West LA.

Prices in the Los Angeles area had also gone down a lot, so we found a great condo in West LA that we could afford, and we bought it. Being back in West LA made my work life a whole lot easier. We stayed there about five years, until I took a job in Riverside.

When we listed the condo, the LA real estate market was really hot, and it sold quickly for what we thought was an outrageous asking price (more than double what we'd paid for it only five years earlier). So, we went house hunting in Palm Desert and opened escrow on a really cool house that was on a golf course, with a pool. Then two weeks later, the LA condo fell out of escrow. We put it back on the market, and it sold quickly, for even more money, and we heaved a sigh of relief. Then two days later the new buyer canceled. At least this time, we had a backup offer, and the buyer still wanted it. She said she'd been sticking pins into a Voodoo Doll in hopes that the buyers would cancel. So the third time was the charm. We moved to Palm Desert, and life was good for the next seven years, until Alan got sick and died.

But even after we moved to West LA, we were still looking to get out of LA. We'd bought a second home in Big Bear (about a two-hour drive from home) with some of the cash we got out of the Long Beach house. And we bought an all-wheel drive SUV so we didn't have to worry about snowy roads. We'd go up there almost every weekend. Alan would ski and I would stay home and work on the novel I was writing. I'd drop him off in the morning and when he was ready to quit, he'd call me from the top of his last run and I'd pick him up at the bottom.

But that still didn't get us out of LA. At that point, we were focusing on Fort Collins, Colorado. We were planning a visit over Thanksgiving to check it out. Then came 9/11, and we decided that flying anywhere right then probably wasn't a very good idea, so we changed our plans and decided to check out the Sun City retirement community in Phoenix, and the one in Tucson. Phoenix offered the added advantage of our being able to spend a few days with our good friend Paula, who was living there at the time.

On the way to Arizona, we stopped to check out the Sun City in Palm Desert and were very impressed. The houses were less expensive—at least by LA standards—and they were really nice. In addition, they had two golf courses and several beautiful resort-style pools. By the time we left for Arizona, we'd pretty much decided that one of the Sun City communities was the place to retire—they have them all over the country.

Sun City in Phoenix was equally impressive, and the houses were about $100,000 less than a comparable home in Palm Desert. But the one in Phoenix had a couple of major drawbacks. It took about an hour to drive in to Phoenix, and the area it was in didn't have much more to offer other than a lot of big box stores like Home Depot, and fast-food places like McDonald's and Taco Bell. The best restaurant we found in the area was the restaurant in Sun City. Not exactly the kind of area where we were looking to live.

After we'd visited for a couple of days, Paula left for the Thanksgiving holiday, so we stayed at Sun City for a couple of days to try it out. We had Thanksgiving dinner at a very nice restaurant that she'd recommended in Phoenix. Of course, that meant we had to drive an hour or so to get there.

Sun City in Tucson was even less attractive. First of all, it wasn't really a Sun City property—same developer, but much smaller than the Sun City brand, without all the amenities, like golf courses. We explored Tucson, but didn't particularly care for that city either. Paula had recommended another good restaurant for our anniversary celebration. We really enjoyed it, but that was about it for that segment of our trip.

We'd reserved the place in Tucson for three or four days, but left after two. We were able to reserve a place in the Palm Desert Sun City (they rent out small units to people who are considering purchase) for a couple of nights, so we drove back and checked it out a little more thoroughly. Again, we were really impressed, both by Sun City itself, and by its proximity to Palm Desert and the entire Palm Springs area. By the time we left for home, we'd decided that we wanted to move to Palm Desert. We just didn't know when, because it wasn't financially feasible at that point.

I went back home and back to practicing law in LA. I was already working as a contract lawyer for several bankruptcy firms—rather than as a full-time lawyer for one firm—so I had a decent income. But I'd realized that after working as a contract lawyer for a couple of years, law firms still weren't quite ready for lawyers who weren't in the office on fairly frequently. And because the Internet hadn't yet developed to the point where it was easy to simply email a finished document to the office, the way it is now, it was also easier for *me* if I worked in the office and could use all the equipment and staff.

At some point, the two firms I was doing most of my work for were giving me too much work—equal to a full-time job or more. So I had to pick one. I chose Manatt Phelps, one of the best entertainment firms in Los Angeles. The head of the bankruptcy department had come from a big national firm and had been charged with the task of developing a top-notch bankruptcy department at Manatt. She and I hit it off immediately. I became a permanent part-time attorney for the firm. Unfortunately, after I'd been working for her for a couple of years, she came up against a corporate culture that she couldn't tolerate, and she left to start her own small firm.

About a year after she left, Manatt decided it didn't want to use part-time attorneys like me anymore, and I was laid off. I had been talking to my former boss ever since she left Manatt about my going to work for her as soon as she had enough work to keep me busy, so I called her and asked her if she was ready for me yet. I started the next day.

When I was in court with her one day a year or so later, we started talking to Norm Hanover, a bankruptcy attorney from Riverside. When Norm mentioned that he lived in Palm Desert—about seventy miles from Riverside—I said I'd love to move to Palm Desert, but I needed to find a way of making a living. He told me to come talk to him. And the rest, as they say, is history.

The firm he was with turned out to be one of the best law firms in Riverside, and one of only a few good bankruptcy firms in the area. I tested the arrangement out while continuing to live in LA. When I decided it would work on a more permanent basis, Alan and I put our condo on the market and bought a place on the golf course in Sun City Palm Desert. Of course, neither of us played golf, but we had a beautiful view across two fairways and the driving range, and the house had a swimming pool. When our real estate agent was showing houses to us, he'd asked if we wanted a swimming pool. We hadn't thought about it, but we quickly decided that in the hot desert weather, it sounded like a pretty good idea. We had some anxious moments during the process when the LA condo fell out of escrow twice, but in the end, everything worked out just fine.

Even with a seventy-mile trip each way to the office in Riverside, I really enjoyed the practice there. In

LA, I'd been a small fish in a big pond; in Riverside, I was a big fish in a small pond. Everybody in the legal community knew me and respected me, even the four bankruptcy judges. And I was finally able to bring in some cases on my own. In bankruptcy, because you rarely represent the same client more than once, most business comes from referrals from other attorneys. Since I was one of the few good bankruptcy attorneys in the Riverside area, I was able to develop a good network of referrals for some fairly complex cases (still my favorites).

And the success I enjoyed in Riverside finally put my fear that someone would realize I was really stupid to rest. Over the years, there'd been a number of experiences that fostered my fear, including any time I lost in court, and any time that I felt I was in over my head. But all of that gradually disappeared once I moved to Riverside.

After Alan and I moved to the desert, Norm and I carpooled two days a week, and the firm agreed that I could work from home one day a week, so I only had to drive by myself two days a week. That worked out fine until a year or two later when Norm cut back on his time in the office, and we could only carpool one day a week.

Fortunately, it was an easy drive into Riverside. With very little traffic, it took a little over an hour (not bad when judged by LA standards).

When we moved to the desert, I'd belonged to a book club in LA for many years. It had been started by one of my women bankruptcy lawyer friends. When it was started, you had to be at least forty in order to be a member. Over the years, we took in some new members including my friend Paula, when she lived in LA, and Kikanza who'd been a close friend for years. When we moved to the desert, I would drive in to LA for the monthly meetings, leaving after work and driving from Riverside. Then I'd stay overnight with someone— usually the hostess of the meeting—and then drive back to work in Riverside the following morning. That worked great until we moved to Vegas.

Of course, driving from Riverside in to LA in the afternoon rush hour traffic was sometimes a disaster (although sometimes it took me less time that some of the women who had to go from one side of LA to the other in rush hour traffic). It hadn't taken me long to get used to the light traffic of the drive back and forth to Riverside. But as often as not, the traffic from the East LA

Interchange to my destination was horrible (the drive back to Riverside the following morning was just the opposite). Today, I find it very difficult to drive in LA traffic, even on weekends. I doubt that you could pay me enough to ever live there again.

By the time Norm retired completely several years later, I'd changed my arrangement with the firm so that I was back to working on a contract basis, making my time in the office a little more flexible. I stayed with the firm for a total of about eleven years, through Alan's illness and death, and the period of a year or so when I was a single woman. It only ended when Ronald and I moved to Las Vegas.

When we moved, I had three or four active cases that I took with me as my own clients. By then, the Bankruptcy Court *required* that all filings be done online, making my practice from Vegas really easy. And I could generally make court appearances by telephone. I set up a nice home office in our rental condo, and things worked out well with all my clients. I even got paid my full hourly rate (instead of the fraction I'd received when working as a contract lawyer for the firm). I had a good recommendation to a couple of bankruptcy firms in Las Vegas, but I never needed the work, so I never even contacted them. By the time we decided to move back to California, all my cases had come to a successful conclusion, and I was fully retired. The timing was perfect, since I was about to become deathly ill.

While we lived in Vegas, my law practice was only taking about half my time, so I started looking for something else to do. I ended up starting a blog—*Sweet Home Vegas*—directed at people who lived in Vegas. I had a professional website designed and Ronald and I joined a MeetUp group for bloggers. I researched and wrote articles about things like the schools (terrible), local entertainment (fabulous), and places off the tourist map to visit (Springs Preserve). I also took lots of pictures and used them in my blog posts. I never built much in the way of readership, but I had a lot of fun. When I got sick with what the doctor thought was fibromyalgia, I pretty much dropped the blogging. For some reason, I went to my blog one day to find that someone had hijacked it—it had vanished! That was only a couple of months before we left Vegas, so I never tried to find it. Now, of course, the subject matter—Las Vegas—is no longer of any interest to me.

Alan and I lived in Sun City for about seven years. Because I worked full-time, I found it difficult to make friends there. And because I wasn't there during the day, I never got involved in any of the dozens of special-interest clubs in Sun City. Other than yoga once or twice a week, I didn't know anybody. Except for neighbors, of course, and a lot of other dog owners. We walked Pooh Bear in one of the local parks, and dog owners turned out to be a very social group. Of course, I was more likely to remember the dogs' names than their owners' names.

Because of yoga, Alan was a bit luckier in making friends after we moved to Sun City. When we'd been there a few years, he trained to be a yoga instructor. Once he was certified, he started his own class in Sun City. He was very good, and his class was very popular. Although we never socialized with his students much, we did consider them friends.

Carol, one of the other yoga instructors, was an exception. She and her husband became our close friends. They had always hosted an annual Winter Solstice party, and we soon became co-hosts, alternating years between their house and ours. When Alan died in early November, I turned that year's Winter Solstice party into his memorial service. Later on, I hosted another memorial in the LA area for all our friends there.

Carol and I also became good friends. After Alan died, she and I would go out to dinner every couple of months. She and her husband sold their house in Sun City shortly after Ronald and I sold ours, and they moved to Orange County. Because of the distance (neither couple strays very far from home these days), we don't see much of them, but we still stay in touch.

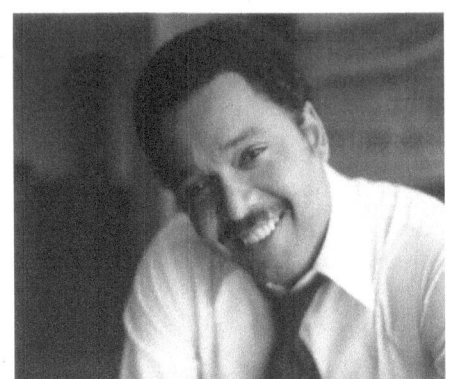

Ronald, 1979

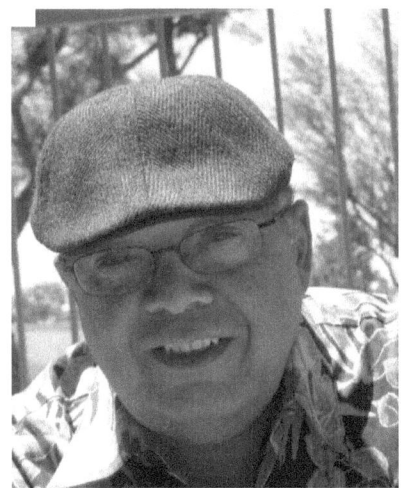

Ronald, 2010

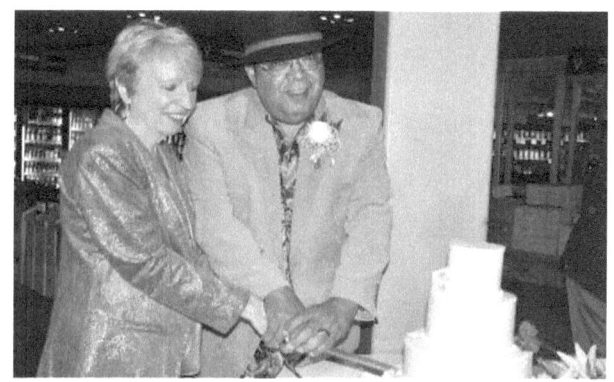

Ronald and Martha wedding, Oct. 31, 2010

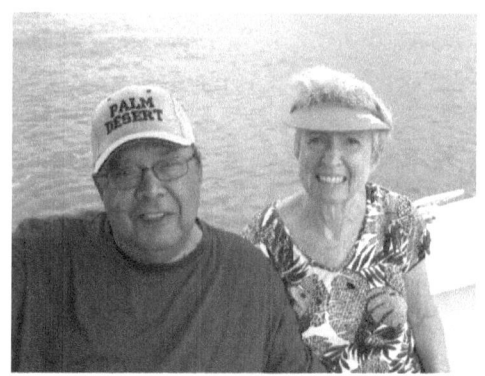

Ronald and Martha sailing in Panama

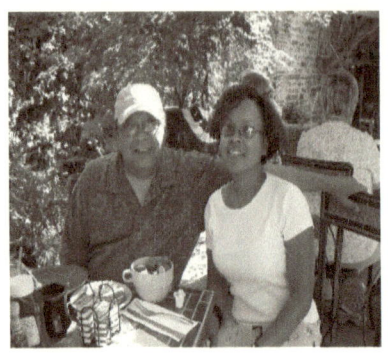

Ronald and Tanya

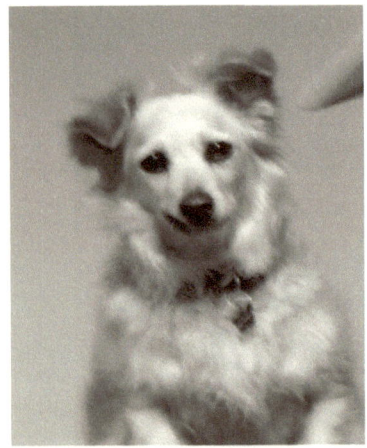

Pooh Bear

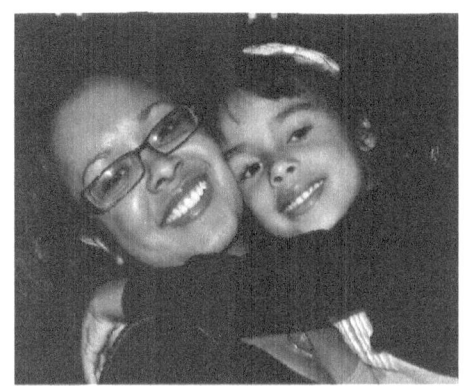

Tanya and Jenny, 2010

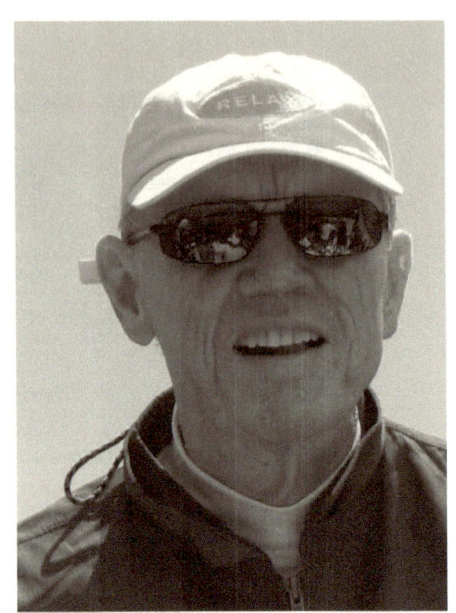

Alan on his sailboat

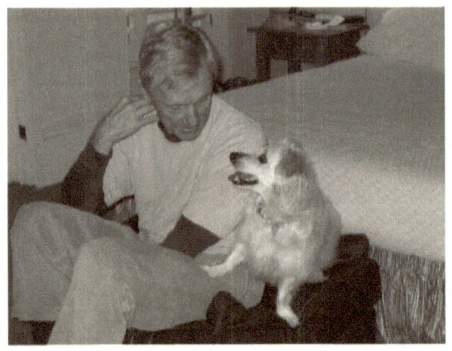

Alan and Pooh Bear

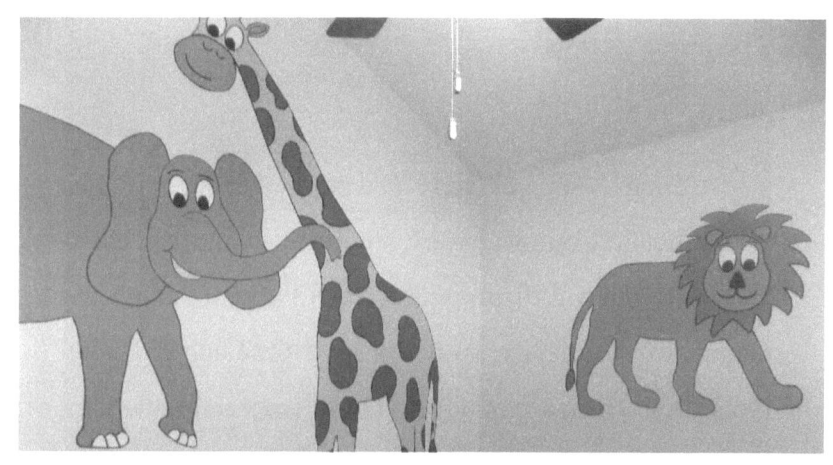

Ronald's office animals

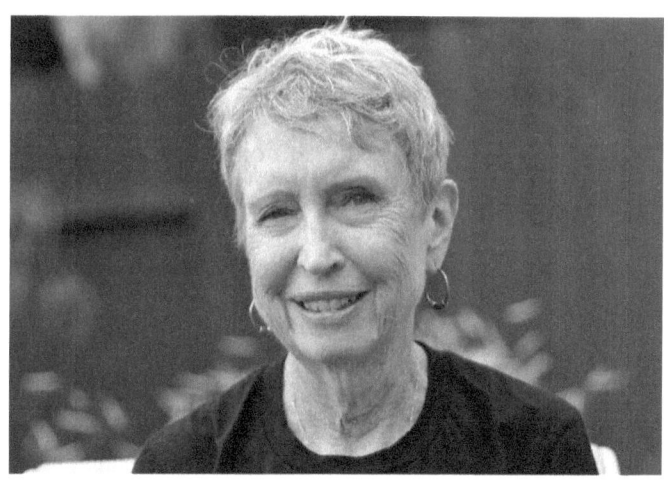

Martha Warriner Jarrett, 2016

Chapter 9

Then Alan got sick. I date the decline in his general health from his bout with prostate cancer in early 2001. Once he was diagnosed, it wasn't urgent that he get treatment immediately, so he took his time and did a lot of research. His main options were surgery and radiation. At his age (nearly seventy), he ruled surgery out pretty quickly. Next, we tried a three-week stay at a place in San Diego that fed you nothing but raw food (someone claimed to have cured their prostate cancer with that treatment). It didn't affect the cancer, but I lost weight (so did Alan, which he certainly didn't need), and all my food sensitivities cleared up. But Alan hated the food—it was supposed to be a healthy diet—but we both quickly grew tired of the heavy doses of wheatgrass.

Because it was supposed to be so healthy, we tried to keep up with the raw-food part once we got home. I bought cookbooks and equipment, including a juicer for wheatgrass and a dehydrator, and there was a local restaurant that served a raw food meal once a week. The restaurant food was fine, but not so much for what I fixed at home. It wasn't an easy method of food preparation, so I would slave over it for an hour or two a day, but when I served it, Alan would say "Yuck" and refuse to eat it. The raw food at home ended pretty quickly. Now, of course, it's quite the rage, and a lot easier to find in restaurants.

In researching the wide variety of available radiation treatments, he decided that the best was a state-of-the-art proton treatment available locally at Loma Linda Medical Center, about an hour from where we lived. The negative was that it wasn't covered by his HMO, so we had to pay for it ourselves. I remember the date clearly; on September 11, 2001, he had to drive out to Loma Linda for treatment. We'd watched the events of that morning on television before he left home, but we still didn't know what was happening, and whether New York and Washington were the only targets. So, he got gas on the way out to Loma Linda and took the daily maximum in cash out of the ATM. I did the same when I went to a court appearance a little later that day. The radiation was an eight-week treatment, and by the end of it, he was already starting to feel poorly. Nothing specific, just not feeling at the top of his game. As the years went by, he just never felt quite well.

During the last few years of his life, it became even worse. He had a bad case of Shingles (his second) after he'd had some minor surgery. That was complicated by some swallowing problems that he'd had for a long time. At one point, it got so bad that I took him to the emergency room because he couldn't even swallow his pain pills. After they shot him full of pain medication and got him calmed down, the doctor said he didn't know whether to admit him to the hospital or not. I urged him to do so, telling him that I didn't know how to take care of him at home. He spent eleven days in the hospital that time.

While he was in the hospital, they did a lot of tests and diagnosed the swallowing problem as achalasia, which is a constriction of the valve that lets food pass from the esophagus into the stomach. They gave him a temporary fix and eventually sent him home. The temporary fix lasted for several years. Then he went in to USC Medical Center in LA and had some sort of balloon inflated in the esophagus. That fix worked until he died a few years later.

During those years, he also got into alternative medicine through a preventive medicine doctor near where we lived. He tried all sorts of things, like chelation therapy (removing the heavy metals from your body), and removing the mercury fillings in his teeth. But any improvement was only temporary. It's from this time that I now suspect he was beginning to suffer from the effects of HIV/AIDS.

One of the things that upsets me now is that the doctor he was going to for all these alternative treatments was in Palm Springs and was involved in gay community health care there. I went to the same doctor for my hormone replacement therapy. After I tested positive for HIV, I called him to see if he had any suggestions for me. But he didn't want to talk to me about anything other than my hormone therapy. I can't help but think that his reaction was based in large part on his sudden realization, when he found out that I was HIV positive, that he'd probably missed something when he was treating Alan around the time of his final illness.

In September 2009, Alan and I took a short cruise down the coast of Mexico. We both got sick. Shortly after we got back—after the antibiotics that we got from urgent care fixed me up but had no effect on Alan—his preventive medicine doctor gave him a couple of doses of antibiotics, as well as some Prednisone, but they didn't seem to help. Then he sent Alan to a specialist—a rheumatologist, I think—because his inflammation numbers were way up. That doctor was going to be out of town for a while, so he called in an internist to take over. But first he did an extensive history that included the fact that Alan had served in Korea during that war. The new doctor was Korean American, and after he'd reviewed Alan's history, he thanked Alan for his service on behalf of his country. Alan said no one had ever thanked him before. At the end of his examination, the new doctor put him in the hospital.

The hospital was the next building over from the doctor's office, so we walked. We were so happy because it looked like Alan finally had a doctor who'd be able to figure out what was wrong with him and fix it. We even talked about going back to Santa Fe once he was feeling better. It had been several years since we'd been there, and it had always been one of our favorite places. But about halfway to the front entrance of the hospital, he ran out of gas and had to sit down. I flagged down someone with an empty wheelchair, and he gave Alan a ride to the admitting desk. They checked him in and took him up to a room. We were both still in good spirits, so I went home.

I'd barely gotten home when I got a call from the doctor telling me that Alan had double pneumonia, and they were putting him on antibiotics. I wasn't particularly worried. The next day, I went to work. About midmorning, I got a call from the doctor telling me that he was putting Alan in intensive care. That's when I freaked. Of course, I was in Riverside, and the hospital was in Rancho Mirage, so it took me close to an hour to get there. Then I couldn't find him. It turned out there were three intensive care units—regular, heart care, and surgical. I finally found him in the heart care section. Guess that was the only bed they had available.

We went along like that for a couple of days, then I got a call in the middle of the night asking me to come to the hospital. When I got there, the nurse told me Alan was fighting his oxygen mask. They'd taken him off the regular oxygen and put him on a pressurized contraption that forced oxygen into his lungs. But it was uncomfortable, so he kept pulling it off. I stayed with him for a couple of hours until he calmed down (with a little help from some drugs), had something to eat, and started using the oxygen all the time. I didn't realize our conversation that night would be the last one we'd ever have.

As I was leaving to go home to get some sleep, the doctors told me they were going to put him on a ventilator in the morning. Now I was really upset. I told them I wanted to see him in the morning to talk to him, but I got there too late. By the time I saw him, he was hooked up to a breathing tube and sedated to the point where he wasn't conscious.

I worked at home for a couple of days so I could visit more often. I held Alan's hand and talked to him, hoping that somehow he knew I was there. I talked to a friend of mine who'd been in an induced coma and had recovered, so I was somewhat encouraged. Alan's doctor talked to me every day and gave me a progress report. Unfortunately, the report was that there was no progress. The antibiotics weren't working. He kept trying different ones, but none of them helped. Neither HIV nor AIDS were never mentioned.

After about ten days, they tried weaning Alan off the ventilator by reducing his sedation and lowering the oxygen. After about half an hour, he was having trouble breathing, so they turned the sedation and the oxygen back up. But during that half hour, he could communicate a little by shaking or nodding his head. I started talking to him and asking him questions. When I was satisfied that he really understood what I was saying, I asked him if he wanted to keep fighting, and he shook his head no.

When I got back to my car, I was pretty upset. I called Maddy to tell her what had happened and to let her know I thought it was time to end his suffering. She agreed that she didn't want him to suffer, but she wasn't quite ready to pull the plug—God, I hate that phrase. So, next I talked to Alan's doctor. He also recommended that I wait a little longer. He had a few more things he wanted to try, so I agreed. About a week later, he told me nothing was working and that there wasn't anything more he could do. Of course, I already knew what I thought should be done. The doctor finally agreed. I called Maddy and her brother Wayne and told them. Maddy agreed, but she wanted to be there. We set a time the following morning.

I had spent many days visiting him—often twice a day—so I was used to him lying there on the bed, not moving. He had the white things around his legs that inflate periodically to keep his legs from getting blood clots, and he was in a hospital gown with a thin blanket over him. The nurses shaved him periodically—but not very well—so he had stubble in various clumps on his cheeks and chin. They used dry shampoo to wash his hair and they'd tried to brush his teeth. All in all, it was very disheartening.

After two weeks on the ventilator, they had to do surgery to take out the breathing tube down his throat and replace it with a tube inserted through an opening in his throat. I thought surgery at that point was an unnecessary indignity, but apparently there was no real choice. I sat in the waiting room and cried until he was out of surgery. I couldn't help but think that the best thing would have been for him to not make it through the surgery. But he did. They returned him to ICU and hooked him back up to the ventilator.

Maddy and her other brother David, whom Alan hadn't seen in years, finally arrived the next morning at the appointed time and the nurses unhooked the ventilator while I waited outside. Then I went in to be with him while he took his final breaths. Maddy and David couldn't handle it, so they waited outside.

It was quite a shock to see him lying there. They'd put tape over the hole in his neck, but nothing could disguise his struggled breathing. It was almost normal for a minute or two, then the breaths started to get farther and farther apart. I held Alan's hand and talked to him. It took fifteen or twenty minutes for him to stop breathing entirely. I kept waiting for him to take another breath. In the end, the next breath never came.

I've had my share of guilt feelings since Alan died. Before I knew what had really killed him, I felt guilty because I thought some of my actions while we were on the Mexican cruise might have contributed to his illness and death. And while I know rationally that I didn't cause his death, on a more emotional level, in the beginning, I wasn't so sure.

Alan died in early November 2009. Before his final illness, my niece, Kathy, in Santa Rosa had offered to do the traditional family Thanksgiving dinner. We didn't want to make the trip, so we declined. Apparently, we weren't alone, so the Thanksgiving gathering was cancelled. After Alan's death, I called Kathy and asked if I could still come. She said sure. Not only did I come, but so did most of my family, including my niece from Chicago.

I left on Monday and drove first to visit my friends near Santa Cruz. It's the longest drive I'd ever made by myself. I drove from Palm Desert, through the LA Basin, and up Highway 5 through the Central Valley. I had the radio and lots of CDs to keep me company. At some point, I turned west and drove through some low hills over to Highway 101 and on to Santa Cruz. About half-way up the grade, I realized I'd forgotten to get gas before I'd turned off the 5. I thought about turning around, but realized that even if I did that, it was five or ten miles from the bottom of the hill until there were any gas stations. I kept going, watching the gas gauge nervously. Finally, I made it over the top of the hill and started down. But it was still at least ten miles before I found a station.

I spent a couple of days with my friends Bob and Gail. Bob was still working, so Gail and I got to do lots of girl things during the day, including lunch at an outdoor restaurant on the Santa Cruz pier and some shopping. We went out someplace nice the first night and cooked dinner the second night.

On Wednesday, I drove up to Kathy's in Santa Rosa. I didn't know until I got there that the whole family would be there. Kathy's husband is a gourmet cook—it was the best Thanksgiving dinner I've ever had. We even had different wine selections for the different courses.

On Friday, Terry and I drove over to Sacramento and spent a couple of nights visiting my brother and his wife. Another good visit. Then I drove home.

Several months later, I received an email from Alan. What? It was one of those email hacks that are directed at friends and family telling them that Alan was supposedly stuck in a foreign country without funds and would someone please wire him some money. I immediately cancelled his email account and changed my email, although even that was hard to do. I only heard from one of his friends that she had received the same email.

The next insult was when I went take his name off one of our credit cards. I wanted to make sure that our reward miles were transferred to my new account. Because he bore all the liability on the account—I could sign on it but the account itself was in his name only— they wouldn't let me transfer the miles. I had to write a letter to somebody in management at the bank and request (politely) that the miles be transferred. Eventually, they were, but I considered it a needless hassle at a very difficult time in my life.

By the time Alan died, I was seeing very little of Maddy. Of course, even when Alan was alive, we didn't see much of Maddy and her family. When we first moved to Palm Desert, they came out to visit us fairly frequently, mainly so the three kids could use the pool, I think. The kids jumped in the pool as soon as they got there, and we had to drag them out for meals. But after a couple of years, they joined a club that had a pool, and that was the last time they visited. Eventually, they bought a house that had a pool, so that really sealed the deal.

Even when Alan and I were living in West LA, and it was only a thirty- or forty-minute drive to their house in La Crescenta, we were doing good to visit them once every three or four months. For one thing, about the only time we were invited to dinner was on Christmas Eve. That was our day for exchanging gifts. But because we weren't invited for Christmas morning—that was Maddy's mother's day—we never got to see the kids open the rest of their presents, especially those that came from Santa Claus.

I'm the one who started the Christmas Eve tradition. Originally, dinner and gifts were at our house, but as the kids came along, it got more difficult for Maddy to pack them up and bring them to our place, so she volunteered to fix dinner instead.

During the last few years of his life, because I didn't want to see him lose his relationship with his daughter altogether, I suggested to Alan that he start inviting himself over at least once a month, and he did. I never went with him. I thought it would be good for Maddy to be able to spend some time alone with her dad. He would drive in from the desert on a Friday afternoon, stay overnight with friends in LA, then visit the kids for a few hours on Saturday morning. I don't think they missed me. Of course, by then the kids were older and usually busy with their own friends. It's nearly impossible to find a time when they're all around.

Once Ronald came back into my life (after Alan's death), it got even worse. I was a bit concerned in the beginning because I thought Maddy and her family might resent him, but the first time we visited them, Maddy's husband said that since Ronald was going to be part of our family, they wanted to get to know him. They even came to our wedding. Obviously, my fears were groundless.

Shortly before Alan's death, I started having some vaginal bleeding, but I ignored it until after he died. Then I made an appointment to find out what was going on. After a bunch of tests that eliminated the possibility of cancer—at least at that point—the verdict was in. I needed a complete hysterectomy. Little surprise there—I'd been avoiding it for years. But the timing was horrible. Plus, I didn't particularly care for my gynecologist in the desert, so I wasn't fond of the idea of his doing my surgery.

One of my friends in my book group had survived ovarian cancer some years earlier, so I decided to try her doctor at Cedars Sinai in LA. Plus, this doctor was married to another of my friends in my book group. I went to see him. He urged me to have the surgery as quickly as possible, so I scheduled it right before Christmas (the day after my memorial for Alan in Palm Desert). As soon as I'd cleaned up from the party, I drove to Maddy's for surgery the following morning.

Since I was having the surgery in LA, Maddy insisted I stay with her until I recovered sufficiently to drive back to the desert. She was a godsend. She drove me to the hospital early the next morning and stayed with me until I was out of surgery and awake. Then she picked me up and took me back to her place the next day. She even called all the people on my list whom I wanted notified after my surgery.

They do surgery now with some kind of advanced robotic device—only three small incisions—so the recovery time is much shorter than it used to be. I was on my feet within two or three days. I stayed at Maddy's until shortly after Christmas. I finally got my chance to share Christmas morning with them and see the kids open their presents.

While I was there, we checked out the place where I wanted to have Alan's LA-area memorial—Descanso Gardens in La Canada. It was beautiful—the banks and banks of camellias were even in bloom. Maddy had to push me around the rough dirt and gravel paths in a wheelchair to check the place out. We set it for January 2, which would have been Alan's seventy-eighth birthday.

I went home for a week, then turned around and drove back to Maddy's on January 2. Wayne had flown in, and we drove to Maddy's together. The memorial went perfectly. My friend Kikanza, from my writing group, officiated. She and I spent a lot of time preparing the service. We used some Native American readings, and some Jewish ones, as well as some standard Christian ones. One of Maddy's friends, whom we'd known for a long time, sang "Amazing Grace." Even David and his wife were there (Alan and his son David had been estranged for years). All our friends from the LA area came. Mary Jo and her husband (of the moment) even drove down from Santa Barbara.

Chapter 10

I started writing about twenty years ago when I joined a writing group of about twelve women. We met at a women's retreat in Santa Fe in the mid-nineties. I was invited by a woman at my gym. We dressed next to each other nearly every day and started talking. She mentioned one morning that she was going to a women's retreat in Santa Fe and would I like to come. Always looking for an excuse to visit Santa Fe, I said sure, even though I didn't know anyone else and I had no idea what would be going on at the retreat. Once we got to Santa Fe, we all hit it off so well that we wanted to find a project we could do together, long-distance. At the end of our three days together, we agreed it would be fun to write a novel. It would be a trashy novel about a professional woman—the kind of book each of us might pick up at an airport for something light to read on a plane. Then we went back to our respective jobs, in various cities across the United States, and didn't think much more about it. Over the next year, however, I took a couple of writing courses so I'd have some idea of what writing a novel might entail.

The next year when we met in Santa Fe, I asked if anyone was still interested. Quite a few were. So, I proceeded to "teach" the rest of the women how to write a novel. At the end of our time together, we agreed to meet in some city every four months. We came up with a main character—Leena Cullen, a mixed-race woman who was looking for a job as director of a museum. We also played with various plotlines, most of which morphed into other ideas over the months and years that followed.

The first group meeting was at my law firm offices in Century City. We started outlining the book and refining the theme. We created a romance, a scandal in Leena's past that would affect her career, and a museum in Washington, DC where she would get a job. We each went home with a homework assignment. None of us, however, worked on any homework assignment—ever.

About four months later, we met again at the Paramount Ranch in Agoura, where a member of our group was a staff writer on *Dr. Quinn, Medicine Woman* (Paramount Ranch is where the popular show was shot). Almost everyone who'd signed up to work on the book was there. We spent three days working on a detailed outline—so detailed that any one of us could write a section of the book by ourselves. It was a process that worked amazingly well for the six or eight years it took us to finish the book.

Over the course of our writing, we met in various places—Los Angeles; Rancho Mirage (where one member had a time-share we used so we could get in a full week of writing); Flagstaff; Washington, DC; Phoenix; and Amherst, Massachusetts. On one of our visits to DC, I played the role of an attorney who was moving to the DC area, and we asked a real estate agent to show us places for sale. We even looked at one in the Watergate. That apartment became the setting for our heroine when she lived in Washington, DC. We wrote, we read what we'd written out loud to the group, and we made changes. But we also had fun—lots of it. Over the years we spent writing the book, we all became close friends.

During the final year, Paula and I took over the major editing chore so that we'd have some hope of actually finishing. When we finally did, everyone read and approved it. The next step was to find an agent. I took on that task but was ultimately unsuccessful. I guess we were a little too forward in our thinking. Our heroine's romantic interest was a black Senator who was thinking about running for president. Sound familiar? Unfortunately, by now it was 2007 or 2008. If only we'd finished a couple of years earlier.

About the time we started writing this book, I started writing a novel of my own. I'd discovered a book called *The Artist's Way* by Julia Cameron, which became my bible. After going through all the book's exercises, I decided I would write a novel—a best-selling one. It would be a legal thriller. I based it on a story I saw in the newspaper about a big corporation that was playing games and concealing relevant documents during litigation.

Another book that I read around that time that had a big influence was *Women Who Run with the Wolves*. It's a series of myths and fables. The one that really resonated with me was the fable of the ugly duckling. I read it and it went *thunk!* As a child, I'd never felt like I belonged. Even as an adult, I never felt that I was a member of the club. When I became a contract partner at Reid & Hellyer (no share of the upside or the downside), I think that feeling finally disappeared. Of course, that feeling probably also went along with my nearly constant fear that people would discover I was really stupid.

Around the time I was reading that book, Alan and I went to Sedona for our anniversary and we found a gorgeous print of a wolf—the head of a wolf in a snowstorm with her (had to be a female wolf) front legs dangling over some kind of ledge and huge snowflakes floating around. Alan bought it for me and had it beautifully framed when we got home. It still hangs in my home.

I worked on my novel—*A Fine Line* was the working title—for several years while my friends and I were continuing to write our joint book. I revised it numerous times and finally declared it done. One of our friends (Alan's and mine) in Sun City had worked in publishing for many years and still had great contacts in the industry. He read it and liked it. He acted as my agent and sent it to his favorite publisher. At least they read it. But they didn't buy it.

I'd never been totally satisfied with the beginning setup of the book. As real-life business scandals—such as Enron and Worldcom—became public, my scenario seemed rather tame in comparison. So, I put the novel in a drawer and forgot about it for several years.

I pulled it out about a year ago and started working on it again. I came up with a new premise for the book and started revising it. Then when Ronald and I were on vacation a few months later, I finally got to the point where I could declare with certainty that Alan had not only infected me with HIV, but that he'd obviously had an extra-marital affair. When I told Ronald, he said, "Why don't you write a book about that?"

It started as a novel, because I thought it would be easier to sell. But several people I respect, including Ronald, our friend in publishing, and a couple of people who teach creative writing, urged me to write it as a memoir instead. So I did. Writing about things that actually happened to me is certainly a lot easier than inventing things. And much more fun.

I rarely thought about writing for the five or six years after I put my novel in the drawer, but I'm really enjoying it now. I am, once again, a writer. In Joan Didion's memoir, *The Year of Magical Thinking*, she talks about how, when she was a teenager, she wanted to edit passages in the books she read. I have conversations in my head now, and I edit them. I also write and edit passages for this book in my head.

I'm also reading lots of memoirs and other books by writers, which influence my writing. Pat Conroy's *Prince of Tides* was recommended in one of my writing courses some years back as a wonderful source of descriptive writing. I often look to it in shaping a well-crafted description. I just finished his last book, *Low Country Heart*, (he died in March 2016) and found his personal stories full of inspiration:

"I search for plunder and inspiration in every book or poem or story I pick up. Other people's books are treasures when stories emerge in molten ingots that a writer can shape to fit his or her own talents. Magical theft has always played an important part of my own writer's imagination."

I've also been inspired by many of the memoirs I've read. They've showed me the simplest and most effective way to structure a memoir. And, of course, I've been inspired by the moving memoirs of other HIV survivors, including Magic Johnson and his wife, Cookie's, Shawn Decker's and Sean Strub's.

In April of last year, our writing group met in Santa Fe after a gap of more than five years. Because it was only a few months after my hospital stay, Ronald didn't want me to travel alone, so he went with me. We really enjoyed had a good time.

While we were there, the group talked about the possibility of doing something with our book, including a "book about the book." The idea of writing the story of twelve women writing a novel together had always intrigued us. How could twelve people write a novel without it sounding like a patchwork quilt? A few people expressed some interest in working on that kind of project, but more than a year has passed since we all went home, and I notice that nobody's done anything. Guess there isn't that much interest, after all. I think we've all moved on with our lives. We did, however, have a lot of fun. We did our usual amount of eating and shopping. The only thing we missed were the massages at Ten Thousand Waves, which had always been a highlight of our weekends together.

We set up another get-together for the following April, but as the time got closer, more and more people dropped out for one reason or another. By the deadline for making hotel reservations, I think there were only three of us who were still able to make it, so we canceled. Hopefully, we'll be able to make it again sometime soon.

Chapter 11

Looking back, it's not surprising that things didn't work out between Ronald and me the first time around. Not only did he not talk to me about his move to Bakersfield and what he expected me to do (I just assumed he was moving there to be with me), but did he expect me to give up my job with Getty and move to Bakersfield? And there were all the other things that couples usually talk about before they get married. Did he want more kids? Did he want me to raise his six-year-old daughter? Looking back now, we both realize it probably wouldn't have worked for very long. And it would have caused wrenching changes in both our lives, as well as the lives of the people around us. Once again, things seem to have worked out for the best.

But that didn't make it easy on me when he left. I had a pretty rough time. I'd often close the door to my office and cry. I imagine the people I worked with thought it was because I was going through a divorce; I never disabused them of that notion. But I knew I needed to do something. I just didn't know what.

Mary Jo was working at Getty at the time, just down the hall from my office. She was active in leading guest seminars for the est Training, and she'd been talking to me about it. I decided it was worth a try. I went down to her office and asked her if there was a guest seminar I could go to sometime soon. She checked and couldn't find one. But, she said, I didn't need to go to a seminar. I could just enroll. She called somebody and enrolled me over the phone. I started that Saturday.

I made it through the Training just fine—no bathroom breaks and all—but it didn't seem to help. One of the major premises of the Training is that "This is it, and I'm satisfied." Well, I definitely wasn't satisfied when I completed the Training. In addition to a broken heart, I was suffering from hypoglycemia, and nothing seemed to be helping. It left me feeling jittery and nervous— something like a caffeine high. I'd been to a couple of doctors who agreed I had hypoglycemia and gave me the standard diet to fix it. But the diet wasn't working. Nothing seemed to be working.

I continued to struggle. One evening I was on a date with a lawyer I'd worked with several years earlier. After dinner, we went back to his house. I started crying and couldn't stop. It freaked him out. But I made it home on my own. The next morning, when I wasn't any better, I called Paul, my ex-husband. He came over and held my hand until I stopped crying and calmed down. But not long after that, I started having thoughts of suicide. I wasn't seriously considering it, but just the thought of it scared me pretty badly.

So, I made an appointment with a psychiatrist. He did two things that helped turn things around. First, he gave me the same diet the other doctors had, but he told me it would take three or four months for it to work. My body had to heal. As long as I knew that, I figured I could handle the three or four months it would take.

And he also gave me antidepressants. I know now that they don't act that quickly, so it wasn't really the drugs that helped, because I snapped out of my funk within two or three days. But *something* had worked. I felt great. I did what any self-respecting girl would do. I went shopping. I had taken a couple of photography classes at UCLA and learned how to develop my own pictures. So, I bought the equipment I needed to do that at home in my bathroom. And I bought some colorful dinner dishes. It did my spirits a lot of good. I made it through the three or four months, and I started to feel better. Much better.

A couple of months later, I took another est course called the Communication Workshop. That's when I really *got* the Training—even the part about "this is it." Not long after that, Paul told me he hadn't seen any difference in me after I did the est Training, but he saw a big difference after I did the Communication Workshop. So, he took the Training. I know it did him a lot of good, too. That's where he met his second wife, Carol. They've been married for more than thirty-five years.

At the time, the est Training was both controversial and notorious. It had been featured in the movie *North Dallas Forty*, and the long hours and lack of bathroom breaks had become infamous. Both were true. At the time, many of the ideas were pretty radical.

Werner Erhard, the founder, was also something of a controversial figure. Before he developed the est Training, he'd been a used-car salesman. He had deserted his family (wife and two or three children) for another woman, and changed his name (from John Paul Rosenberg). The Training he developed probably didn't contain one original idea. He copied from everywhere—Scientology, Dianetics, European and Far Eastern philosophies, and so on. But he did an outstanding job of melding those various concepts into a single package that was easy for people to understand. He even made my old bugaboo existentialism understandable.

And his teachings have withstood the test of time. They are now integrated into numerous self-help books and management courses. And they've strongly influenced the field of personal coaching.

While he once fled the country because of a personal scandal, in recent years, Erhard has lectured on management technology at Harvard Law School, the John F. Kennedy School of Government, and the MIT Sloan School of Management. He is widely credited with the burgeoning recognition of the concepts of transformation and integrity in business and government.

After I finished the Training, I signed up to assist at the local est center. Assisting consisted of a variety of things—working in the office, doing logistics at seminars and Trainings, and calling people to enroll them in the Training, or just to make sure est had graduates' current address. I participated in several panels at guest seminars—usually composed of lawyers—and I even completed the guest seminal leaders' program (although I was never very successful in the guest seminar arena). The agreement you made when you assisted was that you would get more out of it than you put into it. I always did.

I also took seminars—usually one session a week for eight or ten weeks. One that I remember was called (I think) Be Here Now. It was a variation on the "This is it and I'm satisfied" theme—it was about letting both yourself and the world around you simply be the way you are. Over the couple of years before I met Alan, the Training and my participation really helped me get over Ronald. I had several boyfriends; a couple were even semi-serious. By the time I met Alan, I wasn't really looking for a long-term romance—just someone to spend time and have fun with. Funny how things work out when you let go of your agenda of wanting something too much. And all this participation turned out to be better than any dating service I've seen before or since.

Before I took the Training, Mary Jo had been talking about another est course she'd done called the 6-Day. Among other things, it involved rappelling down a mountain. I thought she must be crazy. But a year later, I signed up to do it. The ropes course was just as crazy as it sounded, but most of it turned out to be fun—especially the zip line.

It took place in the summer at the Kirkwood Ski Resort near Lake Tahoe. At the end of the six days, they set up support groups all over the state and encouraged everyone to participate. I joined one in West LA near where I was living. There must have been thirty or forty people at the first meeting. Over the course of the first couple of years, the group settled down to around fifteen or twenty people. It went on that way for a few more years. As time went along, spouses left, and new spouses—including Alan—joined. And it kept going. We met once a month back in those days and had a potluck dinner. And we shared—five minutes each, with someone timing the shares so things wouldn't go on all night.

And we kept going. It's now been over thirty-five years, and we still meet four to six times a year. As far as we know, ours is the longest lasting 6-Day support group of all time. People have moved away, but there's a core group that tries to come at least once a year. Hardly anyone is left in West LA. People come from Bakersfield, Santa Rosa, San Diego, and South Orange County.

As the years have gone by, these people have become some of my closest friends. They were the ones Alan turned to when I was traveling so much. And Ronald turned to them when I was in the hospital. The format has never changed—a potluck dinner (or brunch), followed by five-minute shares. While we're allowed to go over the five minutes (Alan gave notoriously long shares), that's still the target, and someone still times each share. I guess I really did get a lot out of the Training.

Chapter 12

I didn't realize until recently that Ronald also had a pretty rough time of it after he walked out on me. Somehow, I didn't think the person who broke it off, as he had, would suffer in the same way I did, but it turns out that isn't true. Ronald tells me now that he took to his bed and didn't go to work. And he went through some fairly serious therapy. I have no idea what his wife thought about all this.

Ronald's marriage apparently continued to deteriorate. If it hadn't been for his daughter, I think he would have left a lot sooner. But Tanya was very important to him, something I hadn't realized at the time I first knew him. He stayed with his wife until his daughter turned sixteen. When he finally left, his family therapist told him he should fight to take Tanya with him. She was old enough by that time that her opinion would have counted for a lot. But he didn't try. She still gets on him about that.

Fortunately, leaving her behind didn't turn out so badly. She went to college, graduated from Cal Poly San Luis Obispo (cum laude), and became a teacher. She teaches mostly poor white and brown kids in fifth grade here in Bakersfield and loves it, which I'm sure is part of the reason why she's such a good teacher.

She married Rich, whom she'd known in high school, and while they've had their share of bumps in the road, they seem happy now. They have a daughter, Jenny, who's eleven. She's into swimming and wants to get into science and technology—or maybe art.

Other than once at Hooters when our waitress obviously didn't like the fact that Ronald was with a white woman, I've never experienced any prejudice for dating or marrying a black man. These days, at least in California, hardly anyone even notices. And if they do, they never say anything. Even my family.

Of course, that wasn't always the case. When we first knew each other, there were places Ronald wouldn't take me. There was something going on in New Orleans that I thought would be fun to go to, but Ronald refused to take me. Houston—where we spent a fair amount of time—was different. Enough people from outside the south had moved there that we never had any problem, although I imagine it existed somewhere out of my sight.

Ronald really hadn't experienced much of the prejudice that was rampant at the time he was growing up, because he grew up in an area of Tulsa known as the "Black Wall Street." It was solidly middle class, and it was big enough that it was self-sufficient—with black-owned movie theaters, grocery stores, lunch counters, and so on. And while the bus company wasn't owned by blacks, the drivers were all black and didn't enforce the back-of-the-bus rule (the company had been started to provide transportation for the help). He went to an all-black high school, but it was one of the top high schools in the state, even at that time. Then he went to an historically black college—University of Maryland, Eastern Shore.

Probably another reason he never experienced much prejudice as he was growing up was because his mother could easily have passed for white. When she took her kids anywhere, people didn't realize they were related. They probably thought his mother was the maid, out with her charges.

The only story Ronald has told me about his experiences with segregation was one time when he was five and the family took the bus to visit relatives in another state, and they had to sit in the colored section at the back of the bus. There were no seats available, so he stood in the aisle. Of course, at the time, he was too young to understand why he couldn't sit in the empty seats in the front part of the bus. When the bus stopped for a restroom break, he started talking to a white man who'd been on the bus. When the passengers got back on, the man invited Ronald to sit in the empty seat next to him. When the bus driver said he couldn't let Ronald sit in the white section, the man whipped out his passport, showed it to the driver, and said that he was from Israel and Ronald was his nephew. He said that's how people looked in Israel; he wasn't really black. The driver said okay and left them alone. Ronald's written a wonderful story about that adventure and how he decided after the experience that he wanted to be Jewish. I didn't know he could write that creatively.

I, on the other hand, am about as white as you can get. I had red hair (kind of like Charlie Brown's sweetheart) when I was young. And when I was young, I had a temper to match. After ending up in tears a few too many times, I finally realized that the only one who got hurt when I lost my temper was me, so I learned to keep it under control.

As I reached middle age, my hair got darker (medium brown with blonde highlights now—Ronald would like to see it with even more blonde), with pale white skin and blue eyes. I remember that my mother would never let me wear red (now I often wear it). I finally talked her into getting me a red gingham dress with a white pinafore—I must have been six or seven.

But I was still a redhead when I met Ronald. I had a permanent and wore it natural, like an afro. When we were first together, he gave me an afro pic to use. I kept that pic for years, even after I quit wearing my hair that way, because it reminded me of him.

Although I've lost most of the freckles on my face, my arms are still covered with them. The story I was told was that my mother took me to the beach when I was about six months old and put me under an umbrella, thinking that would protect me from the sun. But, of course, it didn't (guess nobody told her about how sun reflects off water). I burned and then I blistered. Then I got sand in the blisters. The next day, she took me back to the beach, where I burned even more. I don't know if that's what caused the freckles, but I'm sure it didn't help.

As a teenager, I wanted a tan, so I used Coppertone (about the only thing available at the time). I now know that the Coppertone is about an SPF 3. But my mother always insisted that I wear zinc oxide on my nose. Since that doesn't sink in, I'd have a white-caked nose. I hated going to the beach with a white nose, so I didn't want to wear it, but I usually did (thank you, Mother). I didn't spend a comfortable day in the sun until sometime in the seventies when I went to Tahiti during what was its

160

winter. I could lie out all day in the sun reading (all the books I had to read before the start of law school), with only Coppertone, and not burn. I was in heaven. I didn't get my first real tan until the summer I was studying for the bar exam, when I could do it the way you're supposed to—fifteen minutes every day.

When I went to SMU in the sixties, it was still segregated. It had a few students from Africa, but no African American students. But in my junior year, they gave a football scholarship to a black kid named Jerry Levias. Toward the end of that year, the rumor that he hadn't made his grades and wouldn't be back the following year went around campus. But it wasn't true— Jerry Levias not only graduated, he went on to have a very successful career in the NFL.

Although I didn't really think of Texas as being in the Deep South, it clearly was. Plus, a large number of the students were from the South. Because there were no African American students at the school, the southern prejudices weren't much in evidence around campus. That is, until Martin Luther King, Jr. came to speak. Then all the fraternity guys drove around in their convertibles waving huge Confederate flags and shouting rebel yells.

I always thought I was fairly liberal when it came to race relations. My first experience came from my mother when I was a small kid. A black family was trying to move into the neighborhood, and somebody was circulating a petition trying to keep them out. My mother even knocked on doors opposing the petition. I learned my views on race from her. Except when she had an issue with my marrying a Catholic (my first husband, Paul), I don't think she had a prejudiced bone in her body.

My first experience with segregation came on a road trip across Texas with my parents when I was around fourteen. We stopped at a service station to use the restrooms. Even then, I was shocked when I saw they had three restrooms—men, women, and colored. I'm not sure which shocked me more, the segregated restrooms, or the fact that black men and women had to share the same restroom.

I hadn't been at college very long before I asked a southern student in my dorm how she could justify segregation and prejudice, and all that it entailed, when the Declaration of Independence said that we are all created equal. Her answer was that southerners considered black people to be something less than human. Again, I was pretty shocked.

I guess I was fairly arrogant on the issue of race when I got to SMU. After all, I didn't think we had any racial problems in Southern California. My senior class in high school, which had a few blacks, had elected a black as senior class president. I was shocked when, while I was home one summer, the Watts Riots erupted. Boy, did that ever knock me down a peg or two. I was pretty quiet on the issue from then on while I was at school.

I was working that summer at Cole of California as an assistant in the junior swimsuit design department. Cole wasn't far from my father's bank branch in Vernon. We were close enough to Watts that we had to change our route to work until the riots ended.

I also think too that people may not see things if they're not looking for them. When I was with Ronald the first time around, I didn't experience any problems when we went together to restaurants or anyplace else. But a friend who was dating a black man about the same time was always complaining that they would often be seated right outside the kitchen and the like. I think she had a problem with what she was doing. I never did.

Ronald is definitely African American in appearance, yet occasionally people say they didn't realize he's black. But then, he's with a white woman. The funniest story comes from our trip to Panama on vacation a few years ago. Starting with the flight attendant on the plane down, everyone thought he was Panamanian, so they expected him to speak Spanish. Even when Ronald answered her in English, she kept speaking Spanish to him. The same thing happened while we were in Panama. They thought he was being arrogant when he wouldn't speak Spanish. I don't speak much Spanish, but I speak a lot more than he does. I finally realized that, because so many black people had been brought into the country to help build the Panama Canal, Ronald really does look a lot like many of the people who live there.

Chapter 13

Thirty years after Ronald left me, when Alan got sick and ended up in the hospital, Ronald and I happened to be in the middle of a string of email correspondence, mostly about politics and the 2008 election, so we were in frequent contact. As Alan got sicker, I turned to Ronald for advice, and cried on his shoulder, figuratively speaking. He asked for my phone number so we could talk. The first time he called, he caught me in the hospital parking lot. I'd just visited Alan and was pretty discouraged. I was struggling with the question of what to do about Alan and whether I should take him off life support. Ronald said that was a question for Alan's doctor and that I should talk to him. So I did.

At the time, Ronald was living in Tulsa, although he'd only recently returned to the city where he grew up. I didn't even know if he was currently married. When he and his first wife finally split up, around 1990, he stayed in Bakersfield for several years. After Occidental Petroleum sold out and he was out of a job, he became a stockbroker, as well as a business reporter for one of the local network affiliates, where he won a couple of Golden Mikes. Several years later, he was offered a job as a professor of entrepreneurship at Florida A&M University in Tallahassee, but he was too broke to buy a plane ticket to get himself there. He called me, and I loaned him the money. He paid me back out of his first paycheck.

Once he left California and moved to Florida in the early nineties, the occasional lunches ended, and I didn't see him again until after Alan died. Our communications were sporadic, at best. Every once in a while, I'd answer my office phone, and it would be Ronald, with some feeble excuse for calling me. He remarried while he was in Florida, but the marriage only lasted five or six years. He was divorced again by the time he came back into my life.

He loved teaching. Says it was his favorite of all the many jobs he's had. He was named Professor of the Year twice. But when it came to doing what was necessary to gain tenure, he didn't do it. When the grace period was up, he left and moved to Baltimore, where his second wife had family. While he was there, he worked on a proposal for a charter school based on some of the business principles he'd been teaching. It was well-received, but ultimately turned down. After that, he wrote a book—*Discovering the Millionaire in Every Child*. He published it with the help of a six-figure grant from the NASDAQ Education Foundation. But the timing was bad—it coincided with a slump in the stock market—so he didn't get the promised marketing support from NASDAQ. He's rewriting and updating it now.

By the time Alan ended up in the hospital, Ronald was retired, with a limited income. But he was still pursuing his dream of saving the world. Obviously, he hasn't succeeded yet, but at the time, it was what got him up in the morning and kept him moving.

Even before Alan got sick, the thought of remarrying if anything ever happened to him had no appeal at all. I couldn't even imagine dating. When our affair started to heat up again shortly after Alan died, I was caught completely by surprise. If it hadn't been for Ronald, I really don't think I would ever have been interested. He was the perfect solution to a problem I didn't even know I had.

We started talking on the phone every day—often for more than an hour. First in the morning—I'd call him while I took the dog for a walk—and again in the evening—usually from the car while I drove home from Riverside. We would also send each other links to YouTube videos of our favorite love songs.

When Ronald came out to visit me for the first time several months later, his plane was a couple of hours late. I waited for him at the Ontario Airport, watching passengers come down the escalator. I knew his flight had landed and that the passengers were on their way to baggage claim, but I didn't recognize him. Not only had he put on a bit of weight, but he was wearing a bulky winter jacket and a cap that did a pretty good job of concealing his face. I will probably never live that one down. Fortunately, he recognized me.

He spent three or four days with me on that trip. I was a little embarrassed about having a boyfriend so soon after Alan died, so we stayed in a hotel near the airport in Ontario, where we were unlikely to be seen by anyone I knew. We had a wonderful time, and both of us knew immediately that this was it. Our love had lasted. When he asked me to marry him, I didn't hesitate. I wasn't about to make the same mistake by turning him down a second time. I was so certain that I even offered to go to Vegas that weekend and get married. I'm glad we didn't do that because we had such a fun wedding, and I wouldn't have wanted to deprive our family and friends of the opportunity to see us get married.

It happened to be Valentine's Day while he was here. We got hamburgers at In- N-Out and took them back to our room. One evening, we went to the local Hooters for drinks. Our waitress was blonde, and fit the Hooters mold perfectly. She practically draped herself all over Ronald and paid no attention to me. But then our regular waitress came back from her break, and took us back as her customers. She was black, and she couldn't have been more rude to both of us. After we left, we realized that she was one of those black women who don't want their black men to date white women. Neither of us had ever experienced that kind of hostility.

Ronald visited me a couple more times, staying for longer and longer periods. By the third visit, I was comfortable enough with the relationship that he stayed at the house with me. That time, we went to Bakersfield so I could meet his daughter, Tanya, son-in-law, Rich, and granddaughter, Jenny. Jenny was dancing in some kind of recital. Fortunately, we all seemed to like each other. I even met Ronald's ex-wife (the first one). I have to say, though, I still can't understand why he'd been attracted to her all those years ago.

I know that Tanya knows Ronald and I go way back, and I assume she knows we had an affair while he was still married to her mother. But I don't know the details of what she knows, and I've never asked. We've become close; closer than Maddy and I ever were.

After about six months, Ronald moved in with me in Palm Desert, where I was living. I really surprised a couple of my old friends who'd lived through the drama of our breakup thirty-some-years before. They couldn't believe I was jumping back into our old relationship so quickly. Mary Jo, my friend from law school, who'd had a lot of bad luck in her own marriages, strongly advised that I get a prenup. But I didn't feel the need. I was that certain this marriage would be forever. I haven't regretted that decision.

We got married on Halloween at Imbibe Wine Bar in Bakersfield, about four months after Ronald moved in with me. We had to postpone the wedding date once. When we checked with the local hotel to make a reservation for our group of guests, we discovered that a local law firm was sponsoring a business conference of some sort that weekend, and all the rooms were already booked. Of course, we could have found another hotel, but when we found out who was speaking at the conference, we decided to pick another date. We really didn't want our wedding to be going on at the same time as people like Sarah Palin and Dick Cheney were speaking nearby. I guess we were afraid they might create bad karma for our wedding. So, we picked a date a couple of weeks later, which happened to be Halloween.

Except for my brother, whose health was failing, my entire family was there, as were most of my friends from the LA area. Even some of Ronald's friends from his life in Bakersfield—including his best man Duncan—were there. We were married by our friend John, a Lutheran minister from San Luis Obispo, and my friend Kikanza from LA. Ronald's granddaughter dressed in her princess costume. My matron of honor was my longtime friend Gail. She'd been the maid of honor at my first wedding (she was the one who fainted), way back in 1969. The wedding was catered by a popular local eatery, Moo Creamery. They made a beautiful cake—banana nut, if I remember correctly. We hired a local jazz musician and a "girl singer." She and his sax were our music. Although they'd never performed it before, they played "our song"—*Just the Way You Are* by Billy Joel—and we danced together for the first time in more than thirty years. Everyone—particularly Ronald and me—had a wonderful time. Both Imbibe and Moo Creamery were fairly new local businesses at the time. When we moved back here a couple of years ago, we were pleased to find that they are both doing really well.

We went to dinner with my family that night, then spent the night at the hotel where everyone was staying. We didn't really have a honeymoon, though we stopped at a wonderful bed and breakfast in South Pasadena for one night on our way back to the desert. We enjoyed the room, the champagne with hors d'ouvres in the evening, and the baked apples at breakfast the following morning.

It's been a wonderful marriage, just as I thought it would be. We have a really good time together—like the first time around. We just enjoy each other. We love talking to each other about anything and everything.

Ronald has always been interested in politics. His views are of the ultraprogressive kind. I'm a progressive, but not quite as far left as he is. The state of politics during the last election cycle has been endlessly frustrating for both of us. How come the people who end up running for president seem to be the least qualified people we can find?

Ronald talks to me endlessly about what's wrong with the country, what's wrong with the people we elect to political office, and on and on. Occasionally—when he talks about the same thing over and over again—I have to remind him that he's preaching to the choir.

Oh, he has his irritating traits, too (nobody's perfect), like getting up in the middle of the night and going into his office to work, or criticizing my parking (usually because I'm too far from the curb). And sometimes I'd like to be a backseat driver, but I'm learning not to say anything. I find that criticizing your spouse is definitely not a good idea. And he talks too softly. People (including me) are always asking him to speak up because they can't hear him. As we drive along, he'll sometimes start reading from the street signs and billboards. Of course, he does so in a soft enough tone that I find myself asking what he just said, as if I would care if I could hear him. He also talks to himself, again in a soft enough voice so that I can't quite hear what he's saying, and I don't know if I should be listening.

And he's crazy—at least some of his ideas are. He seriously thinks he can save the world, and he's always coming up with some nutty concept he thinks will work. Or some test we ought to give to political candidates to establish they're qualified. We were at dinner one night with a couple we'd just met, and after Ronald ran some of these ideas past them, the wife turned to me and asked if he is always this crazy. I assured her that he is. Luckily, I find his craziness to be one of his most endearing qualities.

We also have similar tastes in things like movies, music, food, restaurants—and even houses. When we were looking for our home in Bakersfield, we liked the same thing and totally agreed on which house we should buy. Other things—like sports—we don't always agree on. I like tennis and football; Ronald, not so much, although he knows more about football and basketball than I ever will. I'm a Dodgers fan; he likes the Cubs. We're both voracious readers, although our tastes are completely different. His tend toward nonfiction, particularly with a political bent, or something to do with poverty in America. My tastes go more toward fiction. I've always been a big fan of legal thrillers, like John Grisham; and detective stories, like those by Michael Connelly. But lately, my tastes have turned more serious. I've been on a World War II kick—*All the Light We Cannot See* and *Nightingale*, for example. And as part of the process of writing this book, I've read a lot of memoirs, like Joan Didion's *The Year of Magical Thinking*, and several by people living with HIV, including Cookie Johnson's *Believing in Magic*.

Our marriage is so good that we rarely say "I love you" to each other (which many people say you should do—often) because we *know* we do. At this point I'd say that Ronald is the love of my life. I've never been happier.

Chapter 14

A couple of years after Ronald and I got married, we decided to move to Las Vegas to retire; thank God we picked Vegas instead of some of the other places we'd thought about. It had a much lower cost of living than almost anywhere in California, and the entertainment and restaurant options were endless. Housing prices were at rock bottom after the housing bubble burst, and it wasn't too long a drive to visit his daughter, Tanya, in Bakersfield. We also figured everyone we knew would flock to Vegas to see us, but we couldn't have been more wrong. The few friends and family who came to Vegas while we lived there were too busy gambling and seeing shows to bother visiting us. If we were lucky, they invited us to join them for dinner or a show somewhere on the Strip.

After we'd been in Vegas for a couple of years, we realized it wasn't a forever place for us. It was very difficult to make friends there. We couldn't even find a church we liked. When our lease was up, we moved to Bakersfield to be close to Ronald's family.

The move from Vegas was a disaster. We hired a local company to do the move, but not only did they refuse to move our computers, they left tons of other stuff behind—even some of the boxes *they* had packed. And we had no recourse because Nevada doesn't regulate moving companies. Actually, Nevada doesn't regulate much of anything other than gambling. I was sure glad to get back to California. It may be an expensive place to live, but at least you get something for your money here.

With the wisdom of twenty-twenty hindsight, I'm amazed that I was able to make the drive from Vegas to Bakersfield by myself—I drove by myself so I could be at the new apartment the next morning when the van arrived; Ronald stayed behind to supervise the loading. By this time, we only had one car, so I rented one to drive to Bakersfield. I was supposed to pick up the car at one of the nearby casinos, but the car didn't show up. After a couple of hours, I finally called Enterprise and they picked me up. By this time, I was frustrated and pissed off and not in a good mood to start the long drive. I took the dog with me and stayed the night at Tanya's. The move was only about five weeks before I ended up in the hospital, so my thinking was somewhat muddled and I wasn't in very good shape physically. But I made it safely. Ronald started out the following morning and met me in Bakersfield for lunch.

The van was unpacked before noon and I immediately started missing things. Because I needed my computer for legal work I was still doing at home, we drove back to Vegas the following weekend and loaded up the car. I had turned the power off when we moved, so there was no air conditioning or lights. We tried to find a hotel room, but there was some motorcycle convention in town and everything near us was sold out. We had no choice but to stay in our hot apartment. We wandered around that night with flashlights. A couple of neighbors saw the light and stopped by to make sure we belonged there. There were tons of things in the apartment that wouldn't fit into our car. Although I didn't know that I was sick yet, I knew the thought of packing up and moving all that stuff was overwhelming—and expensive. Fortunately, we had a nice landlord who packed up everything and put it in storage for us.

But then we started missing things. Some things were important, like the vacuum cleaner. Others were more sentimental, like a metal cowboy sculpture Alan and I had bought years before in Santa Fe that had been on our front patio. I hope it landed on someone else's patio, because it didn't make it into our storage locker. For months, every time something was missing, we'd figure it was in storage. It took several months for me to recover enough physically to drive back to Vegas to clean out our storage locker. We loaded up the car and gave whatever we couldn't carry to charity. There was a lot of stuff we never found, like our Keurig coffeemaker. We just had to chalk it up to experience.

By the time we'd settled on Las Vegas as a place to retire, we'd considered—and rejected—a number of other options, including Athens, Georgia and Austin, Texas. But at the top of our list was Panama. All the research I'd done touted Panama as *the* place to retire. It was friendly to Americans, had a stable political system and economic outlook, unemployment was low, it used the US dollar as its currency, and, because of the Canal Zone, there were a lot of Americans living there, particularly retired military. Plus, it had a low cost of living and good medical care and it offered a lot of financial benefits to retirees, like discounts on movies, restaurants, travel, and so on. We decided to check it out.

We spent a week in Panama and a week in Costa Rica, starting out with three days in Panama City at a small bed-and-breakfast. We chatted every morning with other guests, including one retired military man who was in the process of moving to Panama. He was having trouble getting his US bank to transfer his funds to his Panamanian account so that he could pay the deposit on his new place. We met another couple from San Francisco who'd decided to move to Panama and were looking at areas to live.

Once we left the hotel, we'd cross a major thoroughfare at the bottom of the hill into Casco Viejo: the old city. Of course, to get across the street and into Casco Viejo, we had to pass by some pretty poor housing. And as we drove around, we noticed something else interesting: the motorcycle cops all had a second person sitting on the back carrying an Uzi. We began to wonder how safe Panama really was.

Our first night in Panama City, we took a cab to dinner and asked the driver to pick us up afterward. He spoke reasonable English and was quite a character. When he dropped us off after dinner, we arranged for him to pick us up the next morning to take us on a tour of Panama City.

The next morning, we asked him to take us downtown. Instead, he headed in the opposite direction, across the Bridge of the Americas over the Canal. After a nice tour of the area on that side of the Canal, he finally headed downtown. There was a ton of construction going on: buildings, streets, etc. The skyscrapers were fabulous; they reminded us of the Miami skyline. There was even a Trump tower in the shape of a large sail.

We finally figured out that while the driver spoke fairly good English, he didn't understand it very well. So, we just relaxed and let him take us wherever he wanted.

We had lunch in the food court at a huge shopping mall on the first day. It had all the familiar fast food places like McDonald's and KFC, but I wanted to try a local Panamanian place. My Spanish isn't great, but I can count, so I could order from the numbered menu. The food, however, was terrible. After lunch, we wandered around, then stopped for a smoothie. Again, I ordered by the numbers. But then the woman asked me what kind of sugar I wanted (at least I think that was what she was asking). I was stumped. It must have taken us ten or fifteen minutes just to order that smoothie. After a couple of these questions, I finally figured out that if you ordered everything *regular*, you couldn't go very far wrong.

We had a couple of other instances of difficulties with the language, and a couple of horrible meals before we left Panama City. Between the difficulties with the language, problems finding out where to go for things, and just the general feel of the place, we quickly decided that we didn't want to live in a foreign country—too much work! But we continued with our trip.

Once we'd made that decision, of course, we started hearing about all the reasons we wouldn't want to move to Panama—crime and violence (even in some of the small towns we visited), and political corruption. And one couple who'd moved to Panama from Costa Rica, then drove back to Costa Rica to visit friends, found they couldn't bring their car back into Panama without a permit that they didn't know they needed and didn't have. And it was difficult to get mail. You had to rent a post office box in Miami and mail would be forwarded from there. We met one couple that was ready to move back to the states because it had taken so long to get a new vacuum cleaner.

You couldn't even pay your bills by mail; you had to go to the utility or whatever and stand in line.

We already knew that Costa Rica had a lot of problems—everybody had gates around their property, and bars on all the windows. And the president of Costa Rica had been brought up on corruption charges. We also heard about problems with medical care there, particularly one couple who'd used their retirement savings to build a house in the San Jose suburbs, but had to return to the US when one of them got sick. The final straw, of course, came when they couldn't sell the house in Costa Rica.

But we still had a great vacation. Our destination the first day out of Panama City was El Valle de Ancon, a small mountain town about an hour away. On the way, we stopped for lunch in one of the beach towns that dot the coast. We spotted a McDonald's and headed for it like homing pigeons. After a couple of mediocre-to-poor lunches, it felt like home. We met an expat couple there and heard about their experiences in Panama; they loved it, but then, they lived in a community of expats—not my idea of living in a foreign country—and were members of a large church community.

El Valle was a delightful village in the mountains. We met a couple of ex-pats who had once lived there. They were very helpful. And we found a wonderful restaurant for dinner that night—Casa de Lourdes, a boutique hotel and restaurant owned by a famous chef from Panama City. We both agree that the meal ranks among the best dining experiences either of us has ever had.

The next day we started out for Boquete, a small mountain town at the west end of the country. Boquete was a beautiful town. It's in the hills about an hour from the coast, so the weather is delightful. If—and that's a big if—we were ever to move to Panama, that would probably be where we'd settle.

When we left Boquete, we had reservations at a small boutique hotel on the water, outside a fishing village, near the town of David; I can't remember the name of the place. A horrible road: ruts, gravel, up-and-down hills, and around bends. The couple who ran it was from South Africa. They'd spent a couple of years sailing from South Africa to Panama, through the canal, accompanied by their teenagers and cats. The hotel had ten or twelve bungalows built down the side of a hill to the water. Beautiful setting. They took us out on their sailboat—the one they'd sailed halfway around the world in—one evening at sunset, and served us wine and hors d'oeuvres. When it was time to leave, we drove in to David, dropped off the rental car, and flew to Costa Rica.

After a night in the outskirts of San Jose, we took off for the Arenal Volcano region in north-central Costa Rica, a very popular area with expats. Another great place to live, if you like Costa Rica. After a couple of nights, we drove back toward San Jose and followed our noses to the beach area, about an hour southwest of the city.

We spent one night in a run-down place right on the beach, listening to the waves, then decided we were ready for some luxury. So, we tried the Marriott a few miles up the coast. It was breathtaking—a huge beachfront resort in typical Marriott style. Before we went in, we agreed we'd be willing to pay up to $250 a night. When we got to the front desk and asked for a room, it turned out that a room with an ocean view was about $150 a night (it was off-season). We took it and spent a wonderful couple of days luxuriating at the resort, often in the pool, which was lined with cobalt blue tile. But at the end of the day, we found that Panamanian people were much more friendly than the Costa Ricans.

When our stay was over, we drove back to San Jose and stayed in the same funny little hotel where we'd spent our first night in the country. The next morning, we turned in our car and went to the airport for our return flight to Panama City. We stayed at the same bed-and-breakfast where we'd stayed our first time in Panama City and went back to the same seafood restaurant where we'd eaten that first night. We caught our flight the next morning without incident.

Then we had to change planes and go through customs in Houston. First, Ronald left his laptop on the plane. As we were heading back to the gate to find it, we ran into the flight crew. They had Ronald's laptop, so that was one crisis averted. Next, however, because of the delay, we nearly missed our connecting flight to LA. Then, when we got to LA at about ten p.m., one of our bags was missing. It was supposed to be on the next flight, in about an hour, so we waited. Then we drove back to Palm Desert, exhausted, and went back to our regular routine.

Chapter 15

So now we're living in Bakersfield. It's the kind of town people make jokes about. It's full of Okies. It's extremely conservative. And it's pretty much a redneck place (I guess that goes with Okies). I never thought I'd want to live here—even back when Ronald first moved here.

But I now find that I actually like living here. I like it a lot. It's a nice size, it's got quite a bit going on, and you can get from one side of town to the other in half an hour or less. We moved because of family, but we've stayed because we like it. Of course, it's also got a few deficiencies, like shopping. There's only one mall, and only one department store—Macy's. Even the Sears has closed. If you're looking for upscale shopping, you pretty much have to go to LA or Santa Barbara. And there's not much in the way of good entertainment either. For most of the big-name acts and for theater, you have to go to LA. There's a bus company that runs tours for things like the Hollywood Bowl, the Music Center, some Dodger games, and so on. But Bakersfield's got a lot of good restaurants.

Basque food is a specialty—we're working our way through the popular ones.

We started out renting a luxury senior apartment for the first year we were here. It was on Scenic River Drive. I used to joke that it was neither scenic nor near a river. But it was very convenient for shopping and restaurants, so we liked the area a lot. When we started looking to buy, we tried to stay in the same general area. We were successful—it's in a planned community called Riverlakes; our house is about a mile west of the apartment.

When Alan died, it was in the middle of a horrible real estate slump following the bursting of the housing bubble, so it took two years until I was finally able to sell our house in Palm Desert to some neighbors on a land-sale contract—halfway between renting and selling. They didn't have enough money for a down payment and couldn't qualify for a loan.

The summer we decided we were ready to buy a house, they were finally able to refinance it and pay off the loan I had made them. The process wasn't without its bumps in the road—there was a tax lien that had to be paid off, and so on—but it was finally approved, and the funds arrived just in time to close escrow on our new house.

With the money from the sale, we treated ourselves to a cruise, then used most of the rest of the money from the sale for living expenses and furniture for the new house. After we downsized when we moved to Vegas, we didn't have enough furniture left to fill the new house, even though it's not all that big. We hired a decorator and really had fun furnishing the place. I figured this was probably the last home we would ever have, and I wanted to enjoy it.

The house isn't big—about 1,400 square feet—but it had been totally renovated by the prior owners, who'd bought it out of foreclosure. It's got an open floor plan, granite counters, and high-end stainless appliances—all the stuff they feature on the home-improvement shows. The bathrooms had also been remodeled. Everything but the bedrooms is tiled with that new kind of tile that looks like wood. But the pièce de résistance for my husband had to be the big animals—a lion, a giraffe, and an elephant— painted on the walls in what has become his office. We told the sellers they'd better not paint over them before they moved or we'd walk away.

We've also landscaped the backyard with drought-resistant plants. It already looks great, but it will just get better as it grows and fills in. We've got lots of flowers—the kind that bloom for a long time—four fruit trees, and a couple of shade trees (at least, they're supposed to provide shade in a few years—not so much right now). The weather in Bakersfield isn't very conducive to backyard entertainment, but we still enjoy the way the yard looks out the windows in the kitchen and the family room.

It's also great having Tanya and her family close by. She was a big help to her father when I was sick. And to Pooh Bear. When I was in the hospital, Ronald boarded him with our local vet for two or three weeks. After I got home, we moved him to Rich and Tanya's. He stayed there for a couple of months until I was able to handle him (Ronald worried that he was strong enough to pull me over, even though he was a pretty small dog, and Ronald was probably right). They have a dog, Jada, who's half German Shepherd. She's a real sweetie, and she fell in love with Pooh Bear. Because he was an alpha dog, he'd boss Jada around, and she'd roll over in surrender. They even slept together.

During that time, we'd go over once a week or so and visit Pooh Bear. One evening, we were sitting on the living-room couch, and Pooh Bear was over in the corner of the kitchen. I called to him, and he came running. He spent the rest of the evening with me on the sofa. He must have thought we didn't love him anymore. He got over that real quick.

It was also the perfect place to leave Pooh when we went out of town. Rich says he still misses him. Then they got a second dog—an older one that had belonged to Rich's parents. It turned out that Sugar was another alpha dog. Pooh Bear growled whenever she got close, so we couldn't leave him with them anymore. It wasn't much of a problem, however, because we didn't go much of anywhere after that.

After a couple of months, Ronald thought I was strong enough, so we brought Pooh Bear home. It was really good to have him back with us. Funny how much you miss pets when they're gone. By then, he was thirteen, and his health was beginning to fail. He could hardly hear, and he couldn't see very well. During the last couple of months of his life, the decline became pretty bad. He ran into things, and had trouble finding the door when he needed to go outside. And when I'd take him for a walk, he would walk along the curb, occasionally falling off into the gutter and getting wet. But his personality never changed. Always the same sweet dog.

On New Year's Day, he was on the couch next to me watching football when he started to have seizures. After about five minutes, the seizures stopped. Then they started again about an hour later. This time, they didn't stop. We took him to the emergency vet, and the news wasn't good. They had to heavily sedate him just to get the seizures to stop so they could examine him. The vet said it was probably a brain tumor, and there wasn't much they could do. We made the tough decision to put him down. Although I'd known he wouldn't be with us much longer, it didn't make the final decision any easier. He left us a few days before his fourteenth birthday.

Chapter 16

One of the biggest shocks following my diagnosis was the high cost of my HIV medications. The first time I filled the prescription for my antiretroviral meds, the co-pay was almost $800. The pharmacist checked before filling it to make sure I understood how much it was going to cost. Then I had trouble even getting a refill. We'd been so upset with my care from Kaiser that we changed insurance and doctors as soon as we could. I had a month's worth of meds when we made the switch, but I couldn't get an appointment to see my new doctor soon enough. Finally, I went to urgent care.

The first question the doctor there asked me was what my viral load was. I told him I didn't know, but actually, I had no idea what he was even talking about. I guess my research hadn't been all that good. He gave me a prescription for my meds and got me an appointment with my primary care doctor for the following week.

I went home, did some more research, and found out that there are two blood tests that indicate the level of your HIV infection: viral load and CD4. A normal viral load is zero. HIV drives that number through the roof, as into the hundreds of thousands. I eventually found out that my viral load had been off the charts. It's now down to virtually zero, which means that while I still have HIV, it can't be detected and can't be transmitted.

CD4 is a measure of your immune function. Normally it is 500 or above. When I was in the hospital, mine measured less than 50. They say that 200 is the line between HIV and AIDS. They also say that if you fall below the line for AIDS, you can't come back. That's obviously not true, because my CD4 is now around 400.

So, while I'm not yet totally healthy, and I have to watch out for what they call opportunistic infections, I certainly don't have AIDS. Nor am I ever likely to, so long as I keep taking my meds. Of course, AIDS is no longer the death sentence it once was. Today, there are many people living long lives, even with AIDS.

When I finally got in to see my new primary care doctor, she gave me referrals to see an infectious-disease doctor and a dermatologist, because while I was in the middle of all these other medical problems, a bump on my hand tested positive for cancer, and I'm a redhead, which means I'm always having precancerous lesions taken off.

I also saw a neurologist because I'd had a seizure while I was in the coma. Finally, I got to see the infectious-disease doctor: the primary caretaker for HIV and AIDS patients.

When the doctor walked into the examining room, he said I looked familiar. I shook my head. I certainly didn't know him. He looked at my records, then said he'd seen me while I was in the hospital. The hospital—which wasn't owned by Kaiser and was concerned about the quality of care from the Kaiser doctor—had brought him in to consult on my case. This was the doctor Kaiser wouldn't give a contract to, to treat me.

That explained a lot. While I was in the coma, several of the nurses had come to Ronald crying because they didn't think my doctor was giving me the right kind of care. But when I got out of the hospital, Kaiser sent me to the same infectious disease doctor who'd treated me in the hospital. Their regular infectious disease doctor was out on maternity leave. Neither my husband nor I thought this doctor was very competent. For example, not only did she never explain viral load or CD4 to us, she didn't even tell me what my numbers were. Whatever divine power was guiding us, we certainly made the right decision when we left Kaiser.

Then the doctor started to tell us about some of the things we would be dealing with while I fought my way back to some semblance of health. These were things the doctors at Kaiser had never told us. Then he asked Ronald if he'd been tested. By then, he'd been tested twice. Both tests had come back negative. And he reminded us to practice safe sex. We both laughed. We'd found out we were a bit out of practice when it came to things like condoms. While we tried to use them a couple of times, we never succeeded. By the time I was well enough to really be interested in sex again, we'd learned enough to know that there was a very low risk of my infecting Ronald.

About that time, I started really researching HIV and AIDS. All I knew when I got sick was that there were now medications that allowed you to live a fairly normal life—which the hospital had started me on—and that people my age didn't have to worry about the disease, so nobody tested us for it. My lack of knowledge is typical of the way people think of HIV/AIDS today. Because it's become a manageable disease, it's dropped out of the

196

spotlight. Except for people who are gay, or are in their twenties and thirties and sexually active, people just don't pay much attention to it these days. As I nearly found out, that can be fatal. I'm working with the Kern County Health Dept. and its program to educate people and get them tested.

The HIV/AIDS epidemic in this country goes back at least three or four decades. And while the number of victims is a lot lower today than it was in the early years, it is still a crisis, especially in developing countries. People in this country first became aware of AIDS in the early eighties when it burst on the scene like a nuclear bomb. But decades earlier, it appears to have made the jump from apes to humans, probably in the Belgian Congo. It probably stayed contained in the Congo until 1960, when Belgium withdrew. Faced with a power vacuum, the Congo turned to French-speaking Haiti. Anxious to escape the tyrannical regime of Papa Doc Duvalier, many bureaucrats moved to the Congo to help them establish a working government. While there, it seems that HIV infected the Haitians, who then returned home and started spreading the disease in Haiti. Later in the sixties, Haiti started exporting blood plasma to the US (the sale of plasma was a source of much-needed income for the desperately poor population. Before the plasma was sent to the US, it was all mixed together, making it impossible to tell what plasma was infected and what was not. In any event, this imported plasma was likely one of the early sources of HIV in this country. In those days, of course, no one suspected that the plasma carried a deadly virus, which was yet to be named.

Another event that contributed to the spread of HIV in this country was the Bicentennial Celebration in 1976, when people from all over the world came to our shores to celebrate. Tall Ships from around the world also joined in. Press reports from the time make it clear that there was a lot sex going on between a lot of Americans and people from other countries—both male and female.

Of course, at the time, HIV didn't even have a name, nor was anyone aware of the simmering epidemic. Not until 1984 was it determined that HIV—human immunosuppressive virus—caused AIDS. And it wasn't until 1985 that there was even a test for it. In the next decade, people were dying right and left, particularly gay men. For quite a while, people thought of it as a gay men's disease, so the rest of us didn't worry much about it. And the funding to search for a cure similarly reflected this lack of widespread interest. The Religious Right even saw it as God's punishment for homosexuals' depravity.

In those days, HIV's progress was measured by illnesses, declining CD4 levels, and deaths. The AIDS death rates soared to more than forty thousand a year. With the advent of triple-ARV (antiretroviral) cocktails in 1996, the AIDS deaths tumbled by forty-seven percent between 1996 and 1997. And by 1998, a lot of HIV-positive individuals were still living. They would not have been so fortunate had the mortality rate continued on its previous track.

Until I started doing this research, I'd almost forgotten how devastating the disease was back in the early eighties. After all, I hadn't been directly touched by it. All I knew is what I heard on the news. I didn't realize how difficult it was for the gay community to deal with this unknown terror. For the first several years, nobody knew what it was or how it was transmitted. As a pattern began to emerge, people started to figure out that it was a sexually transmitted disease. But was it a new disease, or an accumulation of the various sexually transmitted diseases that were prevalent among sexually active gay men? At the time, it was hard for gays to talk about it outside their own community because they were afraid heterosexuals would be horrified if they realized how gay men actually had sex. After all, there was little enough help or support for the problem back in those days. Even after people began to realize that condoms might prevent transmission, gays were reluctant to use them because they didn't want to suggest that the man they were about to have sex with might have AIDS. Even gay men didn't want anyone with AIDS to kiss them on the cheek for fear they might get AIDS. In retrospect, all this fear seems like the dark ages.

Then in 1991, a famous heterosexual basketball star named Magic Johnson tested positive for HIV. How had that happened? As years went on, AIDS killed a lot of entertainers, like Rock Hudson, Freddie Mercury, and Eaze-E (not all of them gay). What was going on?

For years, researchers tried to find out where the AIDS virus came from, and how it had turned into a worldwide epidemic. For a long time, it looked like a flight attendant had acquired it somewhere in Africa and spread it to every man he had sex with. And that was a lot of men. Eventually, however, researchers discovered that it had been around a lot longer than that.

They've now established that the virus probably jumped from apes to humans in the late 1800s, and that it slowly advanced across Africa and other countries. The earliest confirmed infection in the United States was in the 1960s or 1970s, although it didn't yet have a name. Although I learned this fact from my research months ago, there are now big headlines about how "Patient Zero," as they called the flight attendant, has now been cleared. They treat it like it's new news.

Today, while it affects much smaller numbers in the United States, AIDS is still a leading cause of death in Africa, and mother-to-child transmission is still the primary cause of infant death in developing countries. Of course, the high rate of infection among the general population in Africa also causes enormous societal problems, many of which result from the death of both parents from AIDS, leaving huge numbers of AIDS orphans, many of whom are also infected.

Many of the HIV diagnoses in this country today are among heterosexuals, although approximately fifty-five percent still result from sex between men. With HIV showing up in so many heterosexual men—often those who were openly promiscuous—or IV-drug users, our original thinking that it was just a gay men's disease has proved tragically wrong. In developing countries, it's also the leading cause of death among women of childbearing age—this is another group that's often ignored. The medical profession's failure to consider possible HIV among older people, who don't fit the current HIV/AIDS profile, has, as seen in my case, also resulted in a more limited tragedy.

By the time Magic Johnson was diagnosed in 1991, the drug companies had developed AZT to treat HIV. Discovered in 1985, it was fast-tracked for testing and became available just twenty-five months later, a record for drug testing at that time.

But let's go back for a minute. From 1981 through 1987, new HIV/AIDS cases and fatalities roughly doubled every year. In 1987 alone, there were more than forty thousand deaths and nearly fifty thousand new cases. Today, there are more than 1.2 million people in the US living with HIV, with 12.8 percent (roughly 156,000) of those unaware that they're infected. Over the last decade, the number of new infections has remained relatively stable, at about fifty thousand new infections per year. But the distribution of the virus has shifted, with the rate among heterosexuals declining, and the number of cases among gay men—particularly gay men of color—increasing.

In 1991, the Centers for Disease Control (CDC) announced that one million Americans were infected. That number now stands at about 1.2 million. In this country, it is largely an urban disease, and while the highest rate of infection is in the northeast, there are also a large number of infections in the south. It is still a leading cause of death among young adults, and it runs rampant in many prisons.

In Kern County, where I live, the cumulative numbers (1981-2015) show a total of 2,906 cases of HIV infection: 11% female, 88% men, 1% transgender. Forty-one percent of the cases are Hispanic, 35% are white, 21% African American; Asian and others are negligible (the Hispanic population in the Kern County is well above the national average; the black population is below-average). Thirty-seven percent of the cases are MSM (sex between men) and IDU (IV drug users), and 12% are heterosexual contact only. I am one of only eight women in the county over sixty-five to be infected (1%). Cases of HIV/AIDS have declined rapidly from the peak in the early nineties, as have deaths. Approximately 1,991 individuals diagnosed with HIV were living in the county as of December 15, 2015; 11% (slightly below the national average) are undiagnosed. Approximately 62% of the cases in Kern County have not had lab tests in the past two years, and are presumed to not be on regular ARV meds. Many of these are among the prison populations of the four high-security prisons in the county.

In the early days, AZT added only about twelve months to the dismal life expectancy of an HIV patient. While the immune numbers originally increased significantly once you started AZT treatment, after about a year, those numbers began to plummet. The side effects of the drug were terrible, and some patients refused to take it. Some long-term survivors believe that if they *had* taken it, they would have soon died.

In 1996, something called the HAART (highly active retroviral therapy) regimen offered hope for improved treatment. It consisted of a combination of several different antiretroviral drugs which decreased a patient's total burden of HIV, maintained function of the immune system, and prevented opportunistic infections that often led to death. But AZT and HAART both had enormous side effects—nausea, diarrhea, diabetes, liver and kidney disease, heart problems, and so on—just like the early retroviral regimens did. These side effects caused many people to refuse treatment. The drug regimen was also byzantine in its complexity.

Originally, HAART offered a complement to the AZT treatment, but today it is the basis for our current antiretroviral regimens. During the years between 2000 and 2010, the treatment became progressively less toxic and easier to take. In 2006, a new therapy that required only one pill a day was introduced. There are more than six such drugs on the market today. My doctor has just switched me to one that's less harmful to my already weakened bones.

The new antiretroviral (ARV) drugs also have the power to block the transmission of HIV. Recent studies have shown that with an undetectable viral load (common among those taking medication on a regular basis), the risk of passing on HIV is virtually zero. In the last couple of years, the inability to transmit the virus has finally caused the number of new cases to start going down dramatically, at least in this country.

There have been many studies regarding the optimal time to start ARV treatment. Originally, it was thought that a patient could take a drug "vacation" when CD4 levels were high, with treatment to be resumed once they dropped. There were also studies that suggested one could delay treatment until CD4 levels dropped. Studies now show, however, that starting treatment when CD4 numbers are still high, and continuing without interruption, is by far the better way to go.

More than 50 percent of those living with HIV/AIDS are now over the age of fifty. Many are long-term survivors who were first diagnosed in the late eighties and early nineties. Others, like me, were over fifty when they acquired HIV. And as we age, we're now facing all the other diseases of aging, such as heart disease, kidney disease, and diabetes. Research indicates that HIV ages the cells faster, and that the normal life expectancy is therefore reduced by about five years, although much of the reduction is likely attributable to other high-risk factors among HIV patients, such as smoking, alcohol, and drugs. And while those of us who survive long enough to experience the effects of aging are glad to be alive, we want more out of life.

Another boon to the HIV/AIDS fight was the introduction in 2012 of Truvada, a drug that is taken by at-risk individuals to prevent getting the HIV virus. It's been wildly successful. The problem, once again, is the cost. Also, getting the at-risk population to take the drug is somewhat difficult—probably a result of our thinking that bad things can't happen to us. There are programs right now in New York and San Francisco that help with the cost (as well as with the cost of antiretroviral drugs) and that try to get the word out. Programs like these are also driving the number of new infections way down. There's also a pre-exposure prophylaxis (PEP) that can be used when one fears exposure, particularly after a sexual assault.

Today, of course, while there is still no cure for HIV or AIDS, thanks to antiretroviral drugs, it has become a largely manageable disease. Antiretroviral drugs, starting with the HAART regimen, became widely available in this country in the late nineties.

The newer drugs are easier to take because they're normally combined in one pill, and because they have substantially fewer side effects. In this country, the main impediment to effective treatment is the cost, which is estimated at approximately $28,000 per year. Even with good medical insurance, the co-pays on these drugs can still amount to well more than many people can afford. Drug companies offer some assistance for those who qualify, AIDS foundations help many acquire the drugs, often for free, and there are state and local programs to substantially reduce the cost, but they're often too short-term and do little to assist middle-income people. Even with good prescription insurance, the co-pays can easily exceed $1,000 a month.

After spending insufficient funds on research in the eighties and nineties (President Reagan refused to even acknowledge HIV/AIDS as a problem), funds have increased dramatically over the last twenty years. But the antiretroviral drugs, which have substantially extended the health and life expectancy of patients diagnosed with HIV, are still not a cure. A cure comes when the virus is not only undetectable, but no antiretroviral medications are required, and the virus can no longer be found anywhere in the body. Although I consider it unlikely, some researchers believe there could be a cure by as early as 2020. But once a cure is discovered, it will likely take years to bring these drugs to market. A vaccine to prevent infection is now in phase 3 testing (it's believed that it will not only prevent infection, but will likely suppress transmission as well), and there's now a once a week injection of an ARV drug (which seems to finally make Charlie Sheen happy). There's now also talk of a matchbook-sized implant that last for six months to a year. The implant should be especially useful in third world countries where it's difficult to get patients to take medicine on a regular basis. In the meantime, the best way of preventing new infections continues to be consistent antiretroviral treatment, and Truvada.

But experts caution against the complacency that seems to have taken hold in this country. Apparently, many people don't take precautions because, after all, all you need to do if you become infected is take one pill a day. But while AIDS is now a manageable disease, it is still a lifelong health challenge. This is not a virus that you want as your companion for the rest of your days.

Chapter 17

Notwithstanding Maddy's comments about her father, I still didn't really understand how I could have gotten this terrible disease at my age—or at any other age. I wanted to find out how many other older women were affected. While information on HIV infections is broken down into men/women, race, and age, the age info is limited to "young people." While that confirmed my initial suspicions that women my age were rarely infected, it didn't do much else. The HIV/AIDS population in the United States continues to be made up mostly of gay men, drug users, young, sexually active straight men, and young women. And while the CDC recommends that everyone between ages thirteen and sixty-four be tested at least once, even that demographic would have left me out.

I guess that's what doctors think, too, because they simply don't test people after about age fifty, even when they can't figure out what's wrong with them. I'd been sick off and on for a couple of years. My doctor in Vegas thought I had fibromyalgia, but that isn't a definitive diagnosis—there's no test for it. She also sent me to a blood doctor when my white cell count was chronically low. He didn't catch it either.

Pretty much the same thing happened with Alan. His physical condition had been deteriorating for a couple of years, but even when he landed in the hospital with double pneumonia that the doctors couldn't cure, no one thought to test him. If they had, they might have saved him, and I'm sure they would have caught mine a lot sooner. Instead, he was on a ventilator for nearly three weeks until I made the tough decision to let him go.

Fortunately, I had a little help from him. As I mentioned earlier, the doctor was able to lower the level of his sedation to a point where Alan could hear me and could nod yes or no to my questions. After I made sure he understood me, I asked if he was ready to go, and he nodded yes. I don't know what I would have done without his guidance. Of course, it took another week for his doctors to give up on his treatment and let me end it. Not a lot of fun.

While my physical recovery took only a couple of months, mentally, my recovery wasn't so quick. My thinking was still a little fuzzy, I could no longer multitask, I couldn't handle stress the way I once had, and I sometimes had trouble remembering things that had happened only ten minutes earlier (of course, that may just be my advancing age).

When Ronald and I first moved back to California from Las Vegas in October 2014, I had to get a new driver's license. I hadn't taken the written test in years, but I'd never had any problem with it, so I didn't bother studying. *Surprised* isn't the word to describe how I felt when I failed the test. Before I tried it again, I tried the practice tests, which they now have online. I couldn't even pass any of them. My Nevada driver's license was still valid, so I didn't worry too much about it. Recently, I tried the practice tests again, and while I missed a few questions, I passed all of them. I took the test again and passed. The feeling of accomplishment that I had after finally passing was like the feeling I'd had when I scored 100% on that chemistry exam all those years ago in college. It was a really big deal!

I've learned that there is a component of HIV that, if untreated for a long time, resembles dementia, so Ronald hadn't been totally off base when he thought that might be what was happening to me. The good news is that when it's caused by HIV, you can recover. Of course, I'll never be able to remember the couple of months or so before I landed in the hospital. I guess that period of my life is gone forever.

But what wasn't so easily fixed was my periodic anxiety. Although I got through the nightmare stage fairly quickly, I kept asking myself, *how did I get here?* and worrying about what would come next. Was I going to get sick and die? I wasn't in denial any longer, but I was having trouble dealing with the situation. My doctor gave me Xanax for my anxiety, but that didn't really handle the problem. I still worried a lot.

I can't describe the tsunami of emotions that I was going through at that time. I still spent a lot of time worrying about what was going to happen. I would lie awake at night picturing all kinds of terrible things.

I tried meditation and yoga. I even read a book about Job from the Bible, hoping to understand why such a horrible thing had happened to me. Magic Johnson's story also inspired me, mostly because of the courage he displayed in talking about HIV so openly back in the day when there was still a lot of stigma associated with it. He even had to face basketball players who didn't want to play with him because they were afraid they might get AIDS from him. It seems pretty silly now, but it was a serious concern at the time. I particularly appreciate what he has accomplished since his diagnosis. He even played in the Olympic Games a year or so later on the first Dream Team. Although I'm sure he's had his low moments, HIV certainly hasn't stopped him. And his story has done enormous good for those who came after him, like me.

Finally, my doctor weaned me off the Xanax and put me on a mild antidepressant. That helped a lot. While I'm not exactly worry free, life finally feels pretty normal. I'm even looking forward to the future. After about eight months, when I thought I felt stable enough, I asked him if I could stop taking the antidepressant. He said yes, and so far, it's been fine. My moments of worry about the future are pretty few and far between.

Chapter 18

Recently, the cost issue jumped up and bit me again. After paying the original $800 co-pay for a couple of months, I tried my insurance company's mail-order service. That reduced the cost to around $100 a month—still high, but manageable. And then, at the beginning of last year, the insurance company increased my co-pay to almost $900 a month, like thousands of others whose medication costs have gone off the charts. I was outraged. We have some retirement savings, so we can manage it, but it's not exactly how I'd like to spend those savings. And what about the people who can't afford it? If I could find a soapbox, I'd get on it about this issue. Of course, there's an easy solution for old people: let Medicare negotiate with the drug companies on prices, like the VA does. But once again, of course, that leaves everyone else struggling to pay for a lifesaving drug. Our health care system is a disaster for which there doesn't seem to be an easy fix. I suppose that some kind of regulation is out of the question with the current climate in Washington, but it's certainly needed. What do we need to do to get

Washington to wake up? How big a stink to we need to make? Do we need a walk on Washington over these ridiculous drug prices? And it's not just HIV meds. What about the EpiPen, or the jerk who bought a drug company and promptly raised the price on a cancer drug by something like 5,000%? Do we need to throw these guys in jail? There *must* be a better way.

After about three months of $900-a-month meds, however, Medicare saved me once again. Another advantage of being old. The $900 a month quickly put me into the so-called donut hole and, almost as quickly, pushed me right through it and back out the other side. So, it seems for eight or nine months out of each year, the costs will go back down to around $100 a month. Thank goodness.

At this point, I've had time to wonder again how I ended up with HIV. While it didn't take long to realize it must have come from Alan, that left the bigger question of where *he* got it. Although I don't really want to know the answer, I'm finally ready to confront the fact that not only did he give it to me, but that he must have been unfaithful. Without reaching that point, I couldn't have written this book.

The next question is, how did the nicest man in the world turn into such a villain? And Alan really did seem like the nicest man in the world. I loved him. Women loved him. I once teased him that if anything ever happened to me, he'd have women lining up with their casseroles, figuring that the way to a man's heart is still through his stomach. He taught yoga, and women flocked to his classes. Some of them even became my friends.

Fortunately or unfortunately—I'm not sure which—it doesn't seem as if I'll ever have an answer to that question.

Chapter 19

These days I'm on a mission to persuade people who fall outside the standard HIV/AIDS profile to get tested. It's all well and good that there *is* a profile. I get it that the profile exists because that's where the bulk of the cases occur. But I want to poke a few holes in that profile so that doctors start to think about the possibility for other patients when they can't figure out what's wrong with those who are obviously very sick. After all, it's just a simple blood test. Most of the stigma that once existed, causing people to hide from the diagnosis, has long since disappeared. There is simply no reason not to test everyone when they get sick with something unrecognizable, particularly since we can now live normal lives on medication. It may be expensive medication, but it's not difficult to get, and certainly not difficult to take. Although it was a tricky regimen back in the days when Magic Johnson was first diagnosed, now it's only one pill a day, every day, for the rest of our lives. Or even a once-a-week injection. And the side effects are minimal.

The other issue I want to bang the drum on is testing a patient's blood. My HIV was strongly suspected when my blood tests in the hospital showed that my immune system was way too low. Once that was discovered, I was tested for HIV. But the test for HIV is not normally included in a standard blood panel, at least in a lot of states, including California, where I live. It requires prior written consent from the patient and I can't imagine that any doctor is going to ask for consent unless they already strongly suspect an HIV infection. If the test was a part of the standard blood panel, a lot more people would be diagnosed in the early stages of the disease before little, if any, damage had been done. Another way, of course, would be to reinstate the mandatory blood tests that used to be required to get a marriage license, and to include HIV in the tests. When I got married the first time, in 1969, everybody had to get a blood test and there was a three-day waiting period before the marriage license was issued. These days, about the only thing they test for is sickle cell anemia, and the only people tested are black couples of child-bearing age. Think of how much better off I would have been if my HIV had been discovered in 2010, when Ronald and I got married, rather than 2014.

I spent the first few months after I got out of the hospital and rehab trying to recover physically. I spent the next eight months or so trying to regain everything else—energy, weight, stamina, mental acuity, and so on. I'm now a little more than two years out, and I think I'm pretty much there. The doctor had to prescribe a liquid supplement to get me to put on some weight, but it worked, at least at first. Then I quit paying attention to my weight until the doctor finally checked and found that I was back down to less than I weighed when I got out of the hospital. I enjoyed eating a few fattening foods—like potato chips—until I got it back up to where I'd like to keep it.

We've got friends we met about eighteen months ago who swear I look much better now than even when they first met me. I also went to Santa Fe about four months after I got out of the hospital, to meet with my writing group. Although I was strong enough to travel, Ronald was uncomfortable letting me travel by myself, so he went with me. But I'm confident I can now handle something like that by myself, without any trouble.

Chapter 20

I've never thought of myself as much of a person of faith. I was raised as a Christian Scientist, but when I was old enough to realize that my parents weren't practicing the basic principle of the religion—no doctors—I looked for another church. I joined the Methodist Church when I was in junior high school, mainly because that's where all my friends went. When I married Paul, who was Catholic, I attended mass with him for most of the nearly ten years we were married. After our divorce, I quit going to church. I didn't even go on Easter Sundays.

It stayed that way until Ronald and I got married. He was raised as a Baptist—his father was a preacher. Once he became an adult, he joined the Unitarian Church, which welcomes anyone, even atheists (Ronald identifies himself as an atheist, but I think he's more like an agnostic). He went to the Unitarian Church when he lived here in Bakersfield years ago, but his wife "got the church" as part of the divorce, so we don't go there now.

So, we've had to search for a church. We tried the Unitarian Church in Las Vegas, but it was in a very bad end of town and looked like a run-down, old single-story house. When we went to visit it, we took one look at it, drove around the block once to take a second look, and turned around and drove home. We tried several other churches while we were in Vegas, including one that was largely gay. We made friends with a couple who went there, but when the wife was diagnosed with pancreatic cancer and went back to San Francisco for treatment, we didn't feel like we really fit in. We tried a few others, but didn't find one that felt right. For the last year or so we were there, we didn't go to church.

Once we moved to Bakersfield, we started looking again. We tried a Unity Church—another independent-thinking place of worship—but it was just too small. Then we tried the local AME church. We liked it, but after a couple of months, when we hadn't made any friends, we moved on.

About that time, we met a couple about our age one day at the movies. When the movie was over, we stood around and chatted for fifteen or twenty minutes. When we realized we were like-minded liberals (a rare breed in Bakersfield), we picked a time and got together. They belong to the Episcopal Church downtown and invited us to join them one Sunday. We've been going there ever since, and have even gotten involved in things like their food bank. And we've made more friends.

My religious beliefs today are not quite as radical as Ronald's. I definitely believe in God, but I'm a little uncertain on some of the rest of religious dogma. Because the Christian Science church believes in a loving God, that is still my perception—none of this fire-and-brimstone stuff. And I believe in Jesus and in miracles (after all I've seen enough of them in my own life).

But I've turned to God in the predicament I now find myself in. It's been very helpful. Even Ronald believes in some sort of divine power, and that things happen when they're supposed to—like our getting back together—and only then.

I feel blessed to have contracted HIV/AIDS at the time I did. Not only did the fact that I discovered my positive status in 2014, rather than the 80s or 90s, save my life, but by the time I was infected, much of the stigma was just a distant memory. Once again, I can't imagine what I might have gone through emotionally if I'd contracted it earlier. In the beginning, I didn't talk about it much. Lots of people knew I'd been very sick, but they were polite enough not to ask what was wrong.

And at the time, I was lonely, fearful and bereft. But as I've gotten stronger, both emotionally and physically, I've been able to talk openly about it. If that hadn't happened, I couldn't have written this book. On the other hand, because there is so little stigma these days, support services are few and far between, particularly in a place like Bakersfield. Because I am strong, however, I did it on my own without too much difficulty—or at least that's the way it feels now.

But now that I have started talking about it, my story is being wonderfully well-received. Comments have ranged from things like "it's a compelling story," "the title is perfect; please don't change it," and even "please don't let anyone discourage you." The artwork for the cover is coming together and I'm excited to get the book done and out there. I've even found a group—Positive Womens Network—that is starting a fellowship that will be training a few women to be HIV/AIDS activists, and I've applied for that.

At this writing, it's been a little over two years since my close brush with death, and I have fully recovered (except for the one pill a day I'll have to take for the rest of my life—unless somebody comes up with a cure). The only remaining physical manifestation is my tongue, which is partially dead—I had a seizure while I was in the hospital and bit through my tongue. Nobody's been able to fix it. Not only does one side of my tongue feel funny, but it's given me a slight speech impediment. Also, I can no longer eat spicy food, which I've always loved.

I've done most of my recovery the hard way—by myself. When we were still with Kaiser, I had one appointment with a psychiatrist. I imagine that if we'd stayed with Kaiser, that would have continued, but we didn't. By the time I saw my new primary care physician, almost three months had passed, and I was over the worst of the emotional upheaval, so I never pressed for a referral.

I've also looked for support services in Bakersfield, and, for the most part, there aren't any. I found a website for one HIV/AIDS group, but when I tried to contact them, they never responded. If you're low income, the county has support services available, but I don't qualify. I recently met a man at church who's an HIV/AIDS counselor with Kern County. Through that contact, I've attended a couple of HIV community meetings, where my story was received with a lot of interest. But otherwise, I've done it all with the support of my husband, friends, and family. Thank goodness for them.

But I *have* made it. I'm off all mood-altering drugs (like Xanax and antidepressants), and I feel really good, although I still have my moments. I realized recently that I haven't finished with the grieving process. Even though I'm happy with my current life, I'm still mourning the life I once had and there are still days when I wonder how in the world all this could have happened to me.

I've recently seen a new definition of forgiveness that really resonated: forgiveness happens when you stop trying to change the past. But the fact that I've forgiven Alan, because I accept what happened and I'm not trying to change it (how stupid would that be?), doesn't mean that I'm not still angry. It's what I think about sometimes when I'm lying awake in the middle of the night and can't go back to sleep. It's what still makes me cry.

And I'm still angry at the universe. I got this disease through no fault of my own, I can't do anything about it, and it will affect me for the rest of my life.

I started writing again about a year ago, and started working on this book last spring. Writing is fun and it's easy. Who knows what I might start writing when I'm done with my memoir. I've already got some ideas.

The cover for the book is symbolic of the lonely journey I've been on. And the title of the book—*A Rough Season*—is similar to the way I felt when I first found out that I'm HIV positive—bereft. It was my rough season.

But at this point, I'm ready to start giving something back. I was an early financial supporter (on a very limited scale) of Aids Project Los Angeles, and I've recently upped my contributions a little. If this book sells, maybe I can up my support a little more. I've also gotten active on Twitter again, following several HIV/AIDS tweets, and occasionally posting messages relevant to my position on getting tested. I just bought a T-shirt that says, "I'm HIV positive, but at least I know where I stand. Do you?" on the front and "Get tested today!" on the back. There's a picture on my web site and I hope to have an opportunity to wear it for book signings and speaking engagements.

But, primarily, I hope to give back to current and future HIV/AIDS patients through the publication of this book. As I said at the beginning, I want my story to serve as a wake-up call to everyone that HIV can come from the most unexpected sources. And the earlier it's diagnosed and treatment is started, the better. So, please, get tested. It doesn't matter how old you are or whether you're in a monogamous relationship. It can come from anywhere.

When you get old, you obviously worry about getting sick and, eventually, about dying. I've worried about all the normal things—cancer, heart attack, and so on. But I was caught completely by surprise when I tested positive for HIV. Never in a million years did I expect something like this to happen to me. And while I nearly died, I have survived. No—I've done more than survive. I've thrived. I not only feel normal physically, but I'm happier than I've ever been.

Thanks to my husband, Ronald, and our wonderful marriage, I'm happier than I ever imagined I could be. I'm now seventy-two years old, so I still think about what's to come—what might get me in the end. But I no longer stress about it. And I no longer worry that it might be HIV/AIDS.

As I struggled through the darkest days after my HIV diagnosis, I began to hear a still small voice—my own. It was telling me that there *is* a light at the end of the tunnel. The light is hope. When all seemed lost, it told me that there is still hope. That I could get through this. And I have. I am finally at peace.

Acknowledgements

In addition to my friends and family, who I acknowledge for their love and support through my ordeal, there are a number of people I want to acknowledge and thank. Some of them are people I know; others are simply people whose contributions to the world of HIV/AIDS and/or writing have inspired me. And still others are the authors of memoirs that have contributed to my efforts in writing *A Rough Season*.

Among my friends and family, I want to thank the following for their love and support: my wonderful husband, Ronald, his daughter Tanya, and our dear friends, Margaret and Nils Carlson. In addition, my family: my niece Terry Ryan, my niece Kathy Tindal, and my sister-in-law, Wanda Warriner. Friends include Paula Van Ness, Carol Morrell, and Kikanza Nuri Robins. And, of course, my Six-Day Group. They've been there for me for over thirty-five years.

My church family at St. Paul's Episcopal Church in Bakersfield has also been a great support—particularly our priest, Tim Vivian. And Jonathan Montalvo, who I met at church, for introducing me to the HIV Community at the Kern County Health Department.

Planned Parenthood for its support and counseling back when I was first diagnosed, and, in particular, Pedro Elias, who is the head of Public Affairs for the Central Valley and beyond, for his encouragement on this project. I look forward to working with him and the whole Planned Parenthood organization on its HIV education and testing program.

In a category by herself is Dyane Filip, who's volunteered her time and artistic services (and those of her daughter Danni) in creating the graphics for my website, cover art, business cards, and so on.

People involved in the HIV/AIDS-world include Magic and Cookie Johnson, Sean Strub (founder of POZ Magazine), Elton John and his foundation, Prince Harry, who's recent public testing for HIV has hopefully inspired others to get tested. Public health figures include Dr. Anthony Fauci, head of infectious disease research at the CDC, numerous people with the Kern County Public Health Dept., my original infectious disease doctor, Sam Raman, and my new doctor, Franco Felizarta, a specialist in infectious disease medicine and Valley Fever.

On the memoir front: Joan Didion, whose memoir *The Year of Magical Thinking*, has influenced all memoir authors who have followed. On my second reading of the book, I even understand what she means by "magical thinking." And who can forget *Eat, Pray, Love* by Elizabeth Gilbert. Also, her recent book on creative writing, *Big Magic: Creative Living Beyond Fear.* And then there's Stephanie Maddow Mack's memoir about her life as Bernie Maddow's daughter-in-law and the months following her husband's suicide; Andie Mitchell's *It Was Me All Along,* about her weight loss of 135 pounds while she was in college and her current food blog about healthy eating. Memoirs about surviving with HIV/AIDS include Cookie Johnson's *Believing in Magic,* her story about life after Magic was diagnosed with HIV (I've read Magic's memoir as well, but it's mostly about his basketball world); Sean Strub, who survived the AIDS epidemic in the gay world of New York City in the 80s and 90s; Shawn Decker, a hemophiliac who acquired AIDS in the Ryan White-era but somehow survived. Even Pat Conroy (whose writing has inspired me for years) tells the story in his *Low Country Heart* of his friend in the nineties who was dying of AIDS, but managed to survive just long enough to receive the benefits of the new AIDS treatments. Also, Cleve Jones, whose memoir inspired the recent ABC mini-series, *When We Rise*, about the Gay Liberation Movement and the HIV/AIDS epidemic.

And then there are those who didn't survive, like Rock Hudson, Eaze-E, (his story was told in the recent movie, *Straight Out of Compton)*, Ryan White, Freddie Mercury of *Queen*, whose recent biography, *Somebody to Love*, weaves his own story together with the history of HIV/AIDS starting with the first evidence of the jump of the simian version of AIDS from chimps to humans around 1908, and its subsequent spread to this country.

On the writing front, there are Julia Cameron and her book, *The Artist's Way* (this book started my writing career back in the 90s), Stephen King's *On Writing*, Pat Conroy, whose book, *Prince of Tides* is the best use of descriptive writing that I've ever seen, and Natalie Goldberg's *Writing Down the Bones.* I'm sure there are many other books that have influenced my writing—I just can't remember all of them. And there's my step-son Jody Summers, who's experiences have paved the way for me in the field of self-publishing. And, of course, Amy

Lusky-Barth, who teaches memoir-writing (among other things) for her counseling and encouragement.

I've also used Kirkus' editing services, for both copy and content. Its editors' help in structuring my book, and advice on which stories to include, and which to discard, were invaluable. Best investment I've ever made. Also kudos to Tim Vandehey and Naren Aryal, whose book, *How to Sell a Crapload of Books*, is my bible on how to promote and sell my book.

www.ingramcontent.com/pod-product-compliance
Lightning Source LLC
Chambersburg PA
CBHW030428290526
45786CB00001B/195